PN Maternal Newborn Nursing
Review Module 8.0

Contributors

Audrey Knippa, MS, MPH, RN, CNE
Nursing Education Coordinator and
  Content Project Leader

Sheryl Sommer, PhD, MSN, RN, CNE
Director, Nursing Curriculum and
  Education Services

Brenda Ball, MEd, BSN, RN
Nursing Education Specialist

Lois Churchill, MN, RN
Nursing Education Specialist

Carrie B. Elkins, DHSc, MSN, PHCNS, BC
Nursing Education Specialist

Mary Jane Janowski, MA, BSN, RN
Nursing Resource Specialist

Sharon R. Redding, EdD, RN, CNE
Nursing Education Specialist

Karin Roberts, PhD, MSN, RN, CNE
Nursing Education Coordinator

Mendy G. Wright, DNP, MSN, RN
Nursing Education Specialist

Chris Crawford, BS Journalism
Product Developer and Editorial Project Leader

Derek Prater, MS Journalism
Lead Product Developer

Johanna Barnes, BA Journalism
Product Developer

Joey Berlin, BS Journalism
Product Developer

Hilary E. Groninger, BS Journalism
Product Developer

Megan E. Herre, BS Journalism
Product Developer

Amanda Lehman, BA English
Product Developer

Spring Lenox, BS Journalism
Product Developer

Robin Nelson, BA English
Product Developer

Joanna Shindler, BA Journalism
Product Developer

Morgan Smith, BS Journalism
Media Developer

Brant L. Stacy, BS Journalism, BA English
Product Developer

Mandy Tallmadge, BS Communication
Product Developer

Karen D. Wood, BS Journalism
Product Developer

Katherine Wood-Raclin, BA English, Mass
Communications
Product Developer

Consultants

Christi Blair, MSN, RN

Beth E. Schultz, MSN, RN

INTELLECTUAL PROPERTY NOTICE

IMPORTANT NOTICE TO THE READER

USER'S GUIDE

Welcome to the Assessment Technologies Institute® PN Maternal Newborn Nursing Review Module Edition 8.0. The mission of ATI's Content Mastery Series® review modules is to provide user-friendly compendiums of nursing knowledge that will:

- Help you locate important information quickly.

- Assist in your remediation efforts.

- Provide exercises for applying your nursing knowledge.

- Facilitate your entry into the nursing profession as a newly licensed PN.

Organization

This review module is organized into units covering antepartum, intrapartum, postpartum, and newborn nursing care. Chapters within these units conform to one of three organizing principles for presenting the content:

- Basic concepts

- Procedures (diagnostic and therapeutic)

- Complications of pregnancy

Basic concepts chapters begin with an overview describing the central concept and its relevance to nursing. Subordinate themes are in outline form to demonstrate relationships and present the information in a clear, succinct manner.

Procedures chapters include an overview describing the procedure(s) covered in the chapter. These chapters will provide you with nursing knowledge relevant to each procedure, including indications, interpretations of findings, client outcomes, nursing actions, and complications.

Complications of pregnancy chapters include an overview describing the complication, followed by risk factors. These chapters will cover data collection, including subjective and objective data, and collaborative care, including nursing care, medications, health promotion, and client outcomes.

Application Exercises

At the end of each chapter there are questions you can use to practice applying your knowledge. The Application Exercises include both NCLEX-style questions, such as multiple-choice and multiple-select items, and questions that ask you to apply your knowledge in other formats, such as short-answer and matching items. After completing the Application Exercises, go to the Application Exercise Answer Key to check your answers and rationales for correct and incorrect answers.

NCLEX® Connections

To prepare for the NCLEX-PN, it is important for you to understand how the content in this review module is connected to the NCLEX-PN test plan. You can find information on the detailed test plan at the National Council of State Boards of Nursing's Web site: https://www.ncsbn.org/. When reviewing content in this review module, regularly ask yourself, "How does this content fit into the test plan, and what types of questions related to this content should I expect?"

To help you in this process, we've included NCLEX Connections at the beginning of each unit and with each question in the Application Exercises Answer Keys. The NCLEX Connections at the beginning of each unit will point out areas of the detailed test plan that relate to the content within that unit. The NCLEX Connections attached to the Application Exercises Answer Keys will demonstrate how each exercise fits within the detailed content outline.

These NCLEX Connections will help you understand how the detailed content outline is organized, starting with major client needs categories and subcategories and followed by related content areas and tasks. The major client needs categories are:

- Safe and Effective Care Environment
    - Management of Care
    - Safety and Infection Control
- Health Promotion and Maintenance
- Psychosocial Integrity
- Physiological Integrity
    - Basic Care and Comfort
    - Pharmacological Therapies
    - Reduction of Risk Potential
    - Physiological Adaptation

An NCLEX Connection might, for example, alert you that content within a unit is related to:

- Health Promotion and Maintenance
    - Ante/Intra/Postpartum and Newborn Care
        - Contribute to newborn plan of care.

Icons

Throughout the review module you will see icons that will draw your attention to particular areas. Keep an eye out for these icons:

 This icon indicates an Overview, or introduction, to a particular subject matter. Descriptions and categories will typically be found in an Overview.

 This icon indicates Application Exercises and Application Exercises Answer Keys.

 This icon indicates NCLEX connections.

 This icon indicates content related to safety. When you see this icon, take note of safety concerns or steps that nurses can take to ensure client safety and a safe environment.

 This icon indicates that a media supplement, such as a graphic, an animation, or a video, is available. If you have an electronic copy of the review module, this icon will appear alongside clickable links to media supplements. If you have a hardcopy version of the review module, visit www.atitesting.com for details on how to access these features.

Feedback

ATI welcomes feedback regarding this review module. Please provide comments to: comments@ atitesting.com.

Table of Contents

Unit 4   Newborn Nursing Care

UNIT 1: ANTEPARTUM NURSING CARE

- Human Reproduction
- Low-Risk Pregnancy
- Complications of Pregnancy

NCLEX® CONNECTIONS

When reviewing the chapters in this section, keep in mind the relevant sections of the NCLEX® outline, in particular:

CLIENT NEEDS: HEALTH PROMOTION AND MAINTENANCE

Relevant topics/tasks include:
- Aging Process
  - Provide care that meets the special needs of the newborn - less than 1 month old.
- Ante/Intra/Postpartum and Newborn Care
  - Assist with fetal heart monitoring for the antepartum client.
- Lifestyle Choices
  - Recognize client need/desire for contraception.

CLIENT NEEDS: BASIC CARE AND COMFORT

Relevant topics/tasks include:
- Nonpharmacological Comfort Interventions
  - Use an alternative/ complementary therapy.
- Nutrition and Oral Hydration
  - Monitor and provide for nutritional needs of client.

CLIENT NEEDS: REDUCTION OF RISK POTENTIAL

Relevant topics/tasks include:
- Alterations in Body Systems
  - Identify signs or symptoms of potential prenatal complication.
- Potential for Complications of Diagnostic Tests/ Treatments/Procedures
  - Identify client response to diagnostic tests/ treatments/procedures.
- Therapeutic Procedures
  - Assist with the performance of a diagnostic or invasive procedure.

UNIT 1	ANTEPARTUM NURSING CARE
Section:	Human Reproduction
Chapter 1	Contraception

Overview

- Contraception refers to strategies or devices used to reduce the risk of fertilization or implantation in an attempt to prevent pregnancy.

- Nurses should determine a client's need/desire for contraception. In addition, a thorough discussion of benefits and risks of each method should be discussed.

- Methods of contraception include natural-family planning, barrier, hormonal, and intrauterine methods, as well as surgical procedures.

- This may be an individual decision or sexual partners may make a joint decision regarding a desired preference.

Natural Family Planning Methods

ABSTINENCE	
Definition	• Abstaining from having sexual intercourse eliminates the possibility of sperm entering a woman's vagina.
Client Instructions	• Refrain from sexual intercourse. This method can be associated with saying "no," but can also incorporate saying "yes" to other gratifying sexual activities such as affectionate touching, communication, holding hands, kissing, massage, and oral and manual stimulation.
Advantages	• Most effective method of birth control • Can eliminate the risk of STIs if there is no genitalia contact
Disadvantages	• Requires self-control
Risks/possible complications/ contraindications	• If complete abstinence is maintained there are no risks.

COITUS INTERRUPTUS (WITHDRAWAL)	
Definition	• Man withdraws penis from vagina prior to ejaculation
Client Instructions	• A male must be able to withdraw the penis prior to ejaculation.
Advantages	• Possible choice for monogamous couples with no other option for birth control, such as those opposed to birth control due to religious conviction
Disadvantages	• Most ineffective method of contraception • No protection against STIs
Risks/possible complications/ contraindications	• Depends on a man's ability to control ejaculation. Adolescent boys frequently lack control to make this an effective method. • Leakage of fluid that contains spermatozoa prior to ejaculation can be deposited in vagina • Risk of pregnancy

CALENDAR METHOD (RHYTHM METHOD)	
Definition	• A woman records her menstrual cycle by calculating her fertile period based on the assumption that ovulation occurs about 14 days before the onset of her next menstrual cycle, and avoids intercourse during that period. Also, taken into account is the timing of intercourse with this method, because sperm are viable for 48 to 120 hr and the ovum is viable for 24 hr.

Client Instructions	• Accurately record the number of days in each cycle counting from the first day of menses for a period of at least six cycles.
	• Determine the start of the fertile period by subtracting 18 days from the number of days in the woman's shortest cycle.
	• Determine the end of the fertile period by subtracting 11 days from the number of days of the longest cycle. For example:
	  ○ Shortest cycle, 26 – 18 = 8th day
	  ○ Longest cycle, 30 – 11 = 19th day
	  ○ Fertile period is days 8 through 19.
	• Refrain from intercourse during these days to avoid conception.

Advantages	• Most useful when combined with basal body temperature or cervical mucus method • Inexpensive
Disadvantages	• Not a very reliable technique • Requires accurate record-keeping • Requires abstinence during fertile periods
Risks/possible complications/ contraindications	• Various factors can affect or change the time of ovulation and cause unpredictable menstrual cycles. • Risk of pregnancy

BASAL BODY TEMPERATURE (BBT)	
Definition	• Temperature will decrease prior to ovulation. This can be used to facilitate conception or be used as a natural contraceptive.
Client Instructions	• Measure oral temperature prior to getting out of bed each morning to monitor ovulation.
Advantages	• Inexpensive, convenient, and no side effects
Disadvantages	• Reliability may be influenced by many variables that may cause inaccurate interpretation of temperature changes, such as stress, fatigue, illness, alcohol, and warmth or coolness of sleeping environment
Risks/possible complications/ contraindications	• Risk of pregnancy

BILLINGS METHOD (CERVICAL MUCUS METHOD)	
Definition	• Fertility awareness method based on ovulation. Ovulation, which is when a woman is most fertile, occurs approximately 14 days prior to the next menstrual cycle. Following ovulation, the cervical mucus becomes thin and flexible under the influence of estrogen and progesterone to allow for sperm viability and motility. The ability for the mucus to stretch between the fingers is greatest during ovulation. This is referred to as spinnbarkeit sign.
Client Instructions	• Engage in good hand hygiene prior to and following assessment. • Begin examining mucus from the last day of the menstrual cycle. • Obtain mucus from the vaginal introitus. It is not necessary to reach into the vagina to the cervix. • Do not douche prior to assessment.
Advantages	• Clients can become knowledgeable in recognizing mucus characteristics at ovulation, and self-evaluation can be very accurate. • Self-evaluation of cervical mucus can also be diagnostically helpful in determining the start of ovulation while breastfeeding, in noting the commencement of menopause, and in planning a desired pregnancy.
Disadvantages	• Some clients may be uncomfortable with touching their genitals and mucus; therefore, the client may find this method objectionable.
Risks/possible complications/ contraindications	• Assessment of cervical mucus characteristics may be inaccurate if mucus is mixed with semen, blood, contraceptive foams, or discharge from infections. • Risk of pregnancy

Barrier Methods

MALE CONDOMS	
Definition	• A thin flexible sheath worn on the penis during intercourse to prevent semen from entering the uterus
Client Instructions	• Place a condom on the erect penis, leaving an empty space at the tip for a sperm reservoir. • Following ejaculation, withdraw the penis from the vagina while holding the rim of the condom to prevent any semen spillage to the woman's vulva or vaginal area. • May be used in conjunction with spermicidal gel or cream to increase effectiveness.
Advantages	• Protect against STIs and involves the male in the birth control method
Disadvantages	• High rate of nonadherence • May reduce spontaneity of intercourse • The penis must be erect to apply a condom • If the penis is withdrawn while still erect, this can interfere with sexual intercourse
Risks/possible complications/ contraindications	• A condom may rupture or leak, thus potentially resulting in an unwanted pregnancy. • Condoms have a one-time usage, which creates a replacement cost. • A condom made of latex should not be used if either partner is sensitive to or allergic to latex. • Only use water-soluble lubricants with latex condoms to avoid condom breakage.
FEMALE CONDOMS	
Definition	• A thin, loose-fitting sheath that is inserted into the vaginal canal during intercourse to prevent semen from entering the uterus. One end is closed with a flexible ring that secures it to the cervix. The outer ring wraps around the external genitalia.
Client Instructions	• Insert it by using the closed-end ring to secure it to the cervix and bring the outer ring to wrap around the labia. • Use oil or water-based lubricant to decrease noise during intercourse.
Advantages	• Protects against STIs
Disadvantages	• High rate of nonadherence • May reduce spontaneity of intercourse

FEMALE CONDOMS	
Risks/possible complications/ contraindications	• May rupture or leak, thus potentially resulting in an unwanted pregnancy • Condoms made of latex should not be used if either partner is sensitive to or allergic to latex. • Only use water-soluble lubricants with latex condoms to avoid condom breakage. • Do not use in conjunction with a male condom.

DIAPHRAGMS AND SPERMICIDES	
Definition	• A dome-shaped cup with a flexible rim made of latex or rubber that fits snugly over the cervix with spermicidal cream or gel placed into the dome and around the rim.
Client Instructions	• Have a provider fit the diaphragm. • Visit a provider to be refitted every two years, if there is a 7 kg (15 lb) weight change, full-term pregnancy, or second-term abortion. • Empty the bladder prior to insertion of the diaphragm. • Prior to coitus, insert the diaphragm vaginally over the cervix with spermicidal jelly or cream that is applied to the cervical side of the dome and around the rim. Keep the diaphragm in place for at least 6 hr after coitus. • Reapply more spermicide with each act of coitus.
Advantages	• Eliminate the need for surgery and gives clients more control over contraception
Disadvantages	• Inconvenient, interfere with spontaneity, and require reapplication with spermicidal gel, cream, or foam with each act of coitus to be effective • Require a prescription and a visit to a health care provider • Must be inserted correctly to be effective
Risks/possible complications/ contraindications	• Not recommended for clients who have a history of toxic shock syndrome (TSS) or frequent, recurrent urinary tract infections • Increased risk of acquiring TSS • TSS is caused by a bacterial infection. Clinical manifestations include high fever, a faint feeling and drop in blood pressure, watery diarrhea, headache, and muscle aches. • Proper hand hygiene aids in prevention of TSS as well as removing diaphragm promptly at 6 hr following coitus. • Diaphragms made of latex should not be used if either partner is sensitive to or allergic to latex.

Hormonal Methods

COMBINED ORAL CONTRACEPTIVES	
Definition	• Hormonal contraception containing estrogen and progestin, which acts by suppressing ovulation, thickening the cervical mucus to block semen, and altering the uterine decidua to prevent implantation
Client Instructions	• This method is in the form of an oral medication that requires a prescription and follow-up appointments with the provider. • Consistent and proper use is necessary for method to be effective • Observe for side effects and danger signs of medication. Signs include chest pain, shortness of breath, leg pain from a possible clot, headache, or eye problems from a cerebrovascular accident, or hypertension. • If one dose is missed, take one pill as soon as possible or with the next dose; if two or three doses are missed, follow the manufacturer's instructions. Use alternative forms of contraception or abstinence to prevent pregnancy until regular dosing is resumed.
Advantages	• Highly effective if taken correctly and consistently • Medication can alleviate dysmenorrhea by decreasing menstrual flow and menstrual cramps. • Reduce acne
Disadvantages	• Do not protect against STIs • May increase the risk of thromboses, breast tenderness, scant or missed menstruation, stroke, nausea, headaches, hormone-dependent cancers, and can be teratogenic • Exacerbate conditions affected by fluid retention such as migraine, epilepsy, asthma, kidney, or heart disease
Risks/possible complications/ contraindications	• Contraindicated for clients with a history of blood clots, cerebrovascular accident, cardiac problems, breast or estrogen-related cancers, pregnancy, smoking, or older than 35 years of age • Effectiveness decreases when taking medications that affect liver enzymes such as anticonvulsants and some antibiotics

PROGESTIN-ONLY ORAL CONTRACEPTIVES	
Definition	• Oral progestins that provide the same action as combined oral contraceptives
Client Instructions	• Take the pill at the same time daily to ensure effectiveness secondary to a low dose of progestin. • Do not miss a pill. • If one dose is missed, take one pill as soon as possible and use another form of birth control for two days; if two doses are missed, follow the manufacturer's instructions. Use alternative forms of contraception or abstinence to prevent pregnancy until regular dosing is resumed. • Use another form of birth control during the first month of use to prevent pregnancy.
Advantages	• Have fewer side effects when compared to a combination of oral birth control pills • Considered safe to take while breastfeeding
Disadvantages	• Less effective in suppressing ovulation than combined oral contraceptives • Increases occurrence of ovarian cysts • Does not protect against STIs • Users frequently report breakthrough, irregular vaginal bleeding, and decreased libido. • Increases appetite
Risks/possible complications/ contraindications	• Effectiveness decreases when taking medications that affect liver enzymes, such as anticonvulsants and some antibiotics.

EMERGENCY ORAL CONTRACEPTIVES	
Definition	• Morning-after pill that prevents fertilization from taking place. It contains progestin.
Client Instructions	• Take pill within 72 hr after unprotected coitus. • Take an over-the-counter antiemetic 1 hr prior to each dose to counteract the side effects of nausea that can occur with high doses of estrogen and progestin. • Have a pregnancy test if menstruation does not begin within 21 days.
Advantages	• Pill is not taken on a regular basis • Can be obtained without a prescription by clients 17 years and older
Disadvantages	• Nausea, heavier than normal menstrual bleeding, lower abdominal pain, fatigue, and headache • Does not provide long-term contraception • Does not terminate an established pregnancy • Does not protect against STIs

EMERGENCY ORAL CONTRACEPTIVES	
Risks/possible complications/ contraindications	• Contraindicated for clients who are pregnant or have undiagnosed abnormal vaginal bleeding

TRANSDERMAL CONTRACEPTIVE PATCHES	
Definition	• Contains norelgestromin (progesterone) and ethinyl estradiol, which is delivered at continuous levels through the skin into subcutaneous tissue.
Client Instructions	• Apply the patch to dry skin overlying subcutaneous tissue of the buttock, abdomen, upper arm, or torso, excluding breast area. • Replace the patch once a week. • Apply the patch the same day of the week for three weeks with no application of the patch during the fourth week.
Advantages	• Maintains consistent blood levels of hormone • Avoids liver metabolism of medication since it is not absorbed in the gastrointestinal tract • Decreases risk of forgetting daily pill
Disadvantages	• Do not protect against STIs • Poses same side effects as oral contraceptives • Skin reaction may occur from patch application
Risks/possible complications/ contraindications	• Same as those of hormonal contraceptives

INJECTABLE PROGESTINS (DEPO-PROVERA)	
Definition	• An intramuscular injection given to a female client every 11 to 13 weeks
Client Instructions	• Start injections the first five days of the menstrual cycle and every 11 to 13 weeks thereafter. • Keep all follow-up appointments. • Maintain an adequate intake of calcium and vitamin D.
Advantages	• Very effective and only requires four injections per year • Do not impair lactation
Disadvantages	• May prolong amenorrhea • Irregular or unpredictable bleeding or spotting • Increases the risk of thromboembolism • Decreases bone mineral density (loss of calcium) • Do not protect against STIs • Should only be used as a long-term method of birth control (greater than two years) if other birth control methods are inadequate

INJECTABLE PROGESTINS (DEPO-PROVERA)	
Risks/possible complications/ contraindications	• The nurse should avoid massaging injection site following administration to avoid accelerating medication absorption, which will shorten the duration of its effectiveness.

CONTRACEPTIVE VAGINAL RINGS (NUVARING)	
Definition	• Contains etonogestrel and ethinyl estradiol that is delivered at continuous levels vaginally
Client Instructions	• Insert the ring vaginally. • Replace the ring after three weeks, and place a new vaginal ring within seven days. Insert the ring on the same day of the week monthly.
Advantages	• Do not have to be fitted • Decreases the risk of forgetting to take the pill
Disadvantages	• Do not protect against STIs • Poses the same side effects as oral contraceptives • Some clients report discomfort during intercourse
Risks/possible complications/ contraindications	• Blood clots, hypertension, stroke, heart attack • Vaginal irritation, increased vaginal secretions, headache, weight gain, and nausea

IMPLANTABLE PROGESTINS (IMPLANON)	
Definition	• Requires a minor surgical procedure to subdermally implant and remove a single rod containing etonogestrel on the inner side of the upper aspect of the arm
Client Instructions	• Avoid trauma to the area of implantation.
Advantages	• Effective continuous contraception for three years • Reversible • May used by mothers who are breastfeeding after four weeks postpartum
Disadvantages	• May cause irregular menstrual bleeding • Does not protect against STIs • Most common side effect is irregular and unpredictable menstruation • Headache
Risks/possible complications/ contraindications	• Increased risk of ectopic pregnancy if pregnancy occurs

INTRAUTERINE DEVICES (IUDS)	
Definition	• A chemically active T-shaped device that is inserted through a woman's cervix and placed in the uterus by a health care provider. Releases a chemical substance that damages sperm in transit to the uterine tubes and prevents fertilization.
Client Instructions	• Requires insertion by a health care provider • Monitor the device monthly after menstruation to assure the presence of the small string that hangs from the device into the upper part of the vagina to rule out migration or expulsion of the device. • Report late or abnormal spotting or bleeding, abdominal pain or pain with intercourse, abnormal or foul-smelling vaginal discharge, fever, chills, a change in string length, or if IUD cannot be located.
Advantages	• Long-term effectiveness • An IUD can maintain effectiveness for one to 10 years • Contraception can be reversed • Does not interfere with spontaneity • Safe for mothers who are breastfeeding • It is 99% effective in preventing pregnancy.
Disadvantages	• May increase the risk of pelvic inflammatory disease, uterine perforation, or ectopic pregnancy • Does not protect against STIs
Risks/possible complications/ contraindications	• Contraindicated in clients who have not had a least one child or are not in a monogamous relationship • May cause irregular menstrual bleeding • A risk of bacterial vaginosis, uterine perforation, or uterine expulsion • Must be removed in the event of pregnancy

Transcervical Sterilization

ESSURE	
Definition	• Insertion of small flexible agents through the vagina into the cervix and fallopian tubes. This results in the development of scar tissue in the tubes preventing conception. • Examination must be done after 3 months to ensure fallopian tubes are blocked
Client Instruction	• Normal activities may be resumed by most clients within 1 day of the procedure.
Advantages	• Quick procedure that requires no general anesthesia • Nonhormonal means of birth control • Essure is 99.8% effective in preventing pregnancy. • Rapid return to normal activities of daily living

ESSURE	
Disadvantages	• Not reversible • Not intended for use in clients during the immediate postpartum period • Delay in effectiveness for three months. Therefore, an alternative means of birth control should be used until confirmation of blocked fallopian tubes occurs. • Changes in menstrual patterns
Risks/possible complications/ contraindications	• Perforation can occur • Unwanted pregnancy can occur if a client has unprotected sexual intercourse during the first three months following the procedure. • Increased risk of ectopic pregnancy, if pregnancy occurs

Surgical Methods

FEMALE STERILIZATION (BILATERAL TUBAL LIGATION SALPINGECTOMY)	
Definition	• A surgical procedure consisting of severance and/or burning or blocking the fallopian tubes to prevent fertilization
Procedure	• The cutting, burning, or blocking of the fallopian tubes to prevent the ovum from being fertilized by the sperm
Advantages	• Permanent contraception • Sexual function is unaffected. • Can be done in the immediate postpartum period
Disadvantages	• A surgical procedure carrying risks related to anesthesia complications, infection, hemorrhage, or trauma • Considered irreversible in the event that a client desires conception
Risks/ possible complications/ contraindications	• Risk of ectopic pregnancy if pregnancy occurs

MALE STERILIZATION (VASECTOMY)	
Definition	• A surgical procedure consisting of ligation and severance of the vas deferens
Procedure	• The cutting of the vas deferens in the male as a form of permanent sterilization

MALE STERILIZATION (VASECTOMY)	
Client Instruction	• Following the procedure, use scrotal support and participate in moderate activity for the next few days. • Be aware that sterility is delayed until the proximal portion of the vas deferens is cleared of all remaining sperm (approximately 20 ejaculations). • Use alternate forms of birth control until the vas deferens is cleared of sperm (usually one to two months). • Follow-up is important for sperm count
Advantages	• A vasectomy is a permanent contraceptive method • Procedure is short, safe and simple • Sexual function is not impaired.
Disadvantages	• Requires surgery • Considered irreversible
Risks/ possible complications/ contraindications	• Complications are rare, but may include bleeding, infection, and anesthesia reaction

View Media Supplement:
- Bilateral Tubal Ligation (Image)
- Spermicides (Image)
- Vasectomy (Image)
- Intrauterine Devices (Image)
- Barrier Method of Contraception-Diaphragm (Image)

Ⓐ APPLICATION EXERCISES

Scenario: A 19-year-old mother of a 4-week-old newborn arrives at the primary care provider's office for a postpartum visit. The nurse reinforces possible birth control options with the client.

1. Which of the following is the best contraception option for the client?

    A. Oral contraceptives

    B. Condoms

    C. Diaphragm and spermicide

    D. Injectable progestins (Depo-Provera)

2. For which of the following forms of contraception should the nurse reinforce the potential for a decrease in bone mineral density with the client?

    A. Intrauterine device (IUD)

    B. Injectable progestin (Depo-Provera)

    C. Transdermal contraceptive patch

    D. Implantable progestin

3. Explain when an emergency oral contraceptive may be taken by the client.

4. A nurse is planning to reinforce teaching regarding permanent birth control methods. Which of the following should be discussed with the client? (Select all that apply.)

    _____ Essure

    _____ Bilateral tubal ligation salpingectomy

    _____ Intrauterine device

    _____ Vasectomy

    _____ Implantable progestin

5. A nurse is reinforcing teaching to a client with a prescription for oral contraceptives about danger signs. Which of the following statements indicates the client needs additional teaching regarding side effects?

    A. "I may experience reduced menstrual flow while using the pill."

    B. "I may develop weight gain during the first few months while taking the medication."

    C. "I may feel out of breath upon rising in the morning until I adjust to the medication."

    D. "I may experience occasional headaches when I start taking the pill."

6. Which of the following should the nurse include when reinforcing teaching to a client about the potential disadvantages of the contraceptive vaginal ring (NuvaRing)? (Select all that apply.)

_____ Amenorrhea

_____ Diarrhea

_____ Vaginal irritation

_____ Weight gain

_____ Increased vaginal secretions

APPLICATION EXERCISES ANSWER KEY

Scenario: A 19-year-old mother of a 4-week-old newborn arrives at the primary care provider's office for a postpartum visit. The nurse reinforces possible birth control options with the client.

1. Which of the following is the best contraception option for the client?

   A. Oral contraceptives

   B. Condoms

   C. Diaphragm and spermicide

   D. Injectable progestins (Depo-Provera)

   The client should be advised of the effectiveness rate of each. An oral contraceptive taken daily or injectable progestin injections taken every 3 months are both good options for the client as both are reversible forms of contraception. The injectable progestin injection has an additional benefit of reducing the occurrence of nonadherence and missed doses, requiring only four injections annually. Condoms and a diaphragm should not be a primary choice because of the high rate of nonadherence, and the incorrect application and insertion respectively. However, if used concurrently with the injectable progestin injections, condoms could offer some protection against sexually transmitted infections.

    NCLEX® Connection: Health Promotion and Maintenance, Lifestyle Choices.

2. For which of the following forms of contraception should the nurse reinforce the potential for a decrease in bone mineral density with the client?

   A. Intrauterine device (IUD)

   B. Injectable progestin (Depo-Provera)

   C. Transdermal contraceptive patch

   D. Implantable progestin

   Depo-Provera has the potential for causing decreased bone density in clients. It is important to educate the client regarding dietary measures such as adding calcium and vitamin D to decrease the likelihood of this occurring. An IUD, transdermal contraceptive patch, and implantable progestin do not decrease bone density in clients.

   NCLEX® Connection: Health Promotion and Maintenance, Lifestyle Choices.

3. Explain when an emergency oral contraceptive may be taken by the client.

   The client may take an emergency oral contraceptive within 72 hr after unprotected coitus.

   NCLEX® Connection: Health Promotion and Maintenance, Lifestyle Choices.

4. A nurse is planning to reinforce teaching regarding permanent birth control methods. Which of the following should be discussed with the client? (Select all that apply.)

   X   **Essure**

   X   **Bilateral tubal ligation salpingectomy**

          Intrauterine device

   X   **Vasectomy**

          Implantable progestin

A vasectomy and bilateral tubal ligation salpingectomy are permanent birth control methods. Essure is irreversible. An intrauterine device and implantable progestin are not permanent means of birth control.

(N) NCLEX® Connection: Health Promotion and Maintenance, Lifestyle Choices

5. A nurse is reinforcing teaching to a client with a prescription for oral contraceptives about danger signs. Which of the following statements indicates the client needs additional teaching regarding side effects?

A. "I may experience reduced menstrual flow while using the pill."

B. "I may develop weight gain during the first few months while taking the medication."

C. "I may feel out of breath upon rising in the morning until I adjust to the medication."

D. "I may experience occasional headaches when I start taking the pill."

Shortness of breath may indicate a pulmonary embolus or myocardial infarction. The nurse should reinforce additional teaching regarding the danger signs of the contraceptives. The other options are all common side effects of oral contraceptives which usually subside after a few months of use or can be alleviated by switching to an alternative brand.

(N) NCLEX® Connection: Health Promotion and Maintenance, Lifestyle Choices.

6. Which of the following should the nurse include when reinforcing teaching to a client about the potential disadvantages of the contraceptive vaginal ring (NuvaRing)? (Select all that apply.)

          Amenorrhea

          Diarrhea

   X   **Vaginal irritation**

   X   **Weight gain**

   X   **Increased vaginal secretions**

The nurse should reinforce client education regarding potential disadvantages of using the contraceptive vaginal ring. These include vaginal irritation, weight gain, and increased vaginal secretions. Amenorrhea and diarrhea are not disadvantages of the contraceptive vaginal ring.

(N) NCLEX® Connection: Health Promotion and Maintenance, Lifestyle Choices.

UNIT 1	ANTEPARTUM NURSING CARE
Section:	Low-Risk Pregnancy
Chapter 2	Prenatal Care

Overview

- Prenatal care is important to promote good outcomes for both mothers and newborns. Providing prenatal care includes gaining an understanding of the physiological changes that occur during pregnancy, establishing a relationship with clients and their families, collecting data, and reinforcing teaching. Nurses must consider cultural practices.

- Prenatal education encompasses a great deal of information provided to a client who is pregnant. Major areas of focus include assisting clients in self-care of the discomforts of pregnancy, promoting safe practices, and fostering positive feelings by the pregnant woman and her family regarding pregnancy and childbirth.

Signs of Pregnancy

PRESUMPTIVE SIGNS	PROBABLE SIGNS	POSITIVE SIGNS
FELT BY THE CLIENT	OBSERVED BY A PROVIDER	CONFIRM PREGNANCY
• Amenorrhea • Fatigue • Nausea and vomiting • Urinary frequency • Breast changes – Darkened areola, enlarged Montgomery's tubules • Quickening – Slight fluttering movements of the fetus felt by a woman, usually between 16 to 20 weeks of gestation • Uterine enlargement • Linea nigra • Chloasma • Striae gravidarum	• Abdominal enlargement related to changes in uterine size, shape, and position • Cervical changes • Hegar's sign – Softening and compressibility of lower uterus • Chadwick's sign – Deepened violet-bluish color of vaginal mucosa secondary to increased vascularity of the area • Goodell's sign – Softening of cervical tip • Ballottement – Rebound of unengaged fetus • Braxton Hicks contractions – False contractions, painless, irregular, and usually relieved by walking • Positive pregnancy test • Fetal outline felt by examiner	• Fetal heart sounds • Visualization of fetus by ultrasound • Fetal movement palpated by an experienced examiner

Serum and Urine Pregnancy Testing

- Pregnancy can be determined by the presence of human chorionic gonadotropin (hCG) or a beta subunit of hCG in the serum or urine. Various tests are available at health care centers or at retail stores for home use. Human chorionic gonadotropin (hCG) may be detectable as early as 7 to 10 days after implantation.

Calculating Delivery Date

- Use Nägele's rule to determine the estimated date of birth (EDB) – take the first day of the woman's last menstrual cycle, subtract three months, and then add seven days and one year. When adding seven days, be sure to use the correct number of days in each month.

Determining Obstetrical History

- Gravidity – Number of pregnancies.

  o   Nulligravida – A woman who has never been pregnant

  o   Primigravida – A woman in her first pregnancy

  o   Multigravida – A woman who has had two or more pregnancies

  o   Parity – Number of pregnancies in which the fetus or fetuses reach viability (approximately 20 to 24 weeks or fetal weight of more than 500 g [2 lb]) regardless of whether the fetus is born alive or not

    ■   Nullipara – No pregnancy beyond the stage of viability

    ■   Primipara – Has completed one pregnancy to stage of viability

    ■   Multipara – has completed two or more pregnancies to stage of viability

- GTPAL acronym

  o   Gravidity

  o   Term births (38 weeks or more)

  o   Preterm births (from viability up to 37 weeks)

  o   Abortions that are elective or spontaneous (prior to viability)

  o   Living children

Data Collection

- Subjective Data

  o   Reproductive and obstetrical history (contraception use, gynecological diagnoses, and prior pregnancies)

  o   Medical history, including the woman's immune status (rubella and hepatitis B)

  o   Family history, such as genetic disorders

  o   Any recent or current illnesses or infections

- ○ Current medications, including substance abuse and alcohol consumption

- ○ Psychosocial history (a client's emotional response to pregnancy, adolescent pregnancy, spouse, support system, history of depression, domestic violence issues)

- ○ Any hazardous environmental exposures; current work conditions

- ○ Current exercise and diet habits

- ○ Desire or goals for birthing process including pain management

- Objective Data

  - ○ Reproductive

    - Ovulation and menses cease during pregnancy

    - Uterine size changes from a uterine weight of 50 to 1,000 g (0.1 to 3 lb). By 36 weeks of gestation, the top of the uterus and the fundus, will reach the xiphoid process. This may cause the pregnant woman to experience shortness of breath as the uterus pushes against the diaphragm.

    - Cervical changes – Chadwick's sign, a purplish-blue color that extends into the vagina and labia. Goodell's sign, marked softening in consistency.

    - The breasts increase in size and the areolas take on a darkened pigmentation

  - ○ Cardiovascular – Change in size and shape of the heart to accommodate increased cardiac output and blood volume (45% to 50% at term) to meet the greater metabolic needs. Heart rate increases during pregnancy. Heart size and shape will return to normal shortly after delivery.

  - ○ Respiratory – Maternal oxygen needs increase. During the last trimester, the size of the chest may enlarge, allowing for lung expansion, as the uterus pushes upward. Increased respiratory rate and decreased total lung capacity.

  - ○ Musculoskeletal – Body alterations and weight increase necessitate an adjustment in posture (lordosis). Pelvic joints relax.

  - ○ Gastrointestinal – Nausea and vomiting may occur due to hormonal changes (in the first trimester) and/or an increase of pressure within the abdominal cavity as the pregnant client's stomach and intestines are displaced within the abdomen. Constipation may occur.

  - ○ Renal – Filtration rate increases during pregnancy secondary to the influence of pregnancy hormones and an increase in blood volume and metabolic demands. The amount of urine produced remains the same. Urinary frequency is common during pregnancy.

  - ○ Endocrine – The placenta becomes an endocrine organ that produces large amounts of hCG, progesterone, estrogen, human placental lactogen, and prostaglandins. Hormones are very active during pregnancy and function to maintain pregnancy and prepare the body for delivery.

- Skin changes
  - Chloasma – Mask of pregnancy (pigmentation increases on the face)
  - Linea nigra – Dark line of pigmentation from the umbilicus extending to the pubic area
  - Striae gravidarum – Stretch marks most notably found on the abdomen and thighs
- Expected vital signs
  - Blood pressure
    - First trimester – Measurements are within the prepregnancy range
    - Second trimester – Diastolic and systolic blood pressure decreases 5 to 10 mm Hg
    - Third trimester – Blood pressure should return to prepregnancy range by term
  - Pulse increases 10 to 15/min around 20 weeks of gestation and remains elevated throughout the remainder of the pregnancy
  - Respirations increase by 1 to 2/min
- Laboratory tests

LABORATORY TEST	PURPOSE
Blood type, Rh-factor, and presence of irregular antibodies	Determines the risk for maternal-fetal blood incompatibility (erythroblastosis fetalis) or neonatal hyperbilirubinemia. For clients who are Rh-negative and not sensitized, the indirect Coombs' test will be repeated between 24 to 28 weeks of gestation.
CBC with differential, Hgb, and Hct	Detects infection and anemia
Hgb electrophoresis	Identifies hemoglobinopathies (sickle cell anemia and thalassemia)
Urinalysis with microscopic examination of pH, specific gravity, color, sediment, protein, glucose, albumin, RBCs, WBCs, casts, acetone, and human chorionic gonadotropin	Identifies diabetes mellitus, gestational hypertension, renal disease, and infection
One-hour glucose tolerance (Oral ingestion or IV administration of concentrated glucose with venous sample taken 1 hr later [fasting not necessary])	Identifies hematuria; done at initial visit for at-risk clients, and at 24 to 28 weeks of gestation for all pregnant women (greater than 140 mg/dL requires follow up)
Three-hour glucose tolerance (Fasting overnight prior to oral ingestion or IV administration of concentrated glucose with a venous sample taken 1, 2, and 3 hr later)	Screens for diabetes mellitus in clients with elevated 1-hr glucose test. A diagnosis of gestational diabetes requires two elevated blood-glucose readings.

LABORATORY TEST	PURPOSE
Papanicolaou (PAP) test	Screens for cervical cancer, herpes simplex type 2, and/or human papillomavirus.
Vaginal/cervical culture	Detects streptococcus ß-hemolytic, Group B (routinely obtained at 35 to 37 weeks of gestation), bacterial vaginosis, or sexually transmitted infections (gonorrhea and Chlamydia).
Rubella titer	Determines immunity to rubella.
PPD (tuberculosis screening), chest screening after 20 weeks of gestation with positive purified protein derivative	Identifies exposure to tuberculosis.
Hepatitis B screen	Identifies carriers of hepatitis B.
Venereal disease research laboratory	Syphilis screening mandated by law.
HIV	Detects HIV infection (The Centers for Disease Control and Prevention and The American Congress of Obstetricians and Gynecologists recommends testing all clients who are pregnant unless the client refuses testing.)
Toxoplasmosis, other infections, rubella, cytomegalovirus, and herpes virus (TORCH) screening when indicated	Screening for a group of infections capable of crossing the placenta and adversely affecting fetal development
Maternal serum alpha-fetoprotein (MSAFP)	Screening occurs between 15 to 22 weeks of gestation. Used to rule out Down syndrome (low level) and neural tube defects (high level). The provider may decide to use a more reliable indicator and opt for the Quad screening instead of the MSAFP at 16 to 18 weeks of gestation. This includes AFP, inhibin-A, a combination analysis of human chorionic gonadotropin, and estriol.

- o   Nursing care
  - ■   At the initial prenatal visit:
    - □   Determine estimated date of delivery using Nägele's rule.
    - □   Obtain medical and nursing history.
    - □   Obtain baseline weight, vital signs.
    - □   Assist with the pelvic examination. Have clients empty their bladder prior to the exam.
    - □   Obtain initial laboratory work.
    - □   Assist with vaginal ultrasound to determine gestational age.

- Listen for fetal heart tones at the midline, right above the symphysis pubis, by holding the stethoscope firmly on the abdomen.

  ‣ Use an ultrasound stethoscope at 10 to 12 weeks of gestation.

  ‣ Use a fetoscope at 16 to 20 weeks of gestation. Listen at the midline, right above the symphysis pubis, by holding the scope firmly on the abdomen. Move the scope across the abdomen until the fetal heart tones are heard. Obtain baseline rate, which should be 110 to 160/min.

- Explain the importance of regular follow-up to include monthly prenatal visits for the first seven months, then every two weeks during the eighth month, and every week during the last month.

 View Media Supplement: Prenatal Interview (Video)

- Ongoing prenatal visits

  - Monitor weight, blood pressure, and urine for glucose, protein, and leukocytes.

  - Monitor for the presence of edema.

  - Monitor fetal development.

  - Listen for fetal heart tones and measure fetal heart rate.

  - Start measuring fundal height after 12 weeks of gestation. Between 18 and 30 weeks of gestation, the fundal height measured in centimeters should equal the week of gestation. Have clients empty their bladder and measure from the level of the symphysis pubis to the upper border of the fundus.

 View Media Supplement: Measuring Fundal Height (Video)

  - Begin assessing for fetal movement between 16 and 20 weeks of gestation.

  - Assist with Leopold's maneuvers to palpate presentation and position of the fetus.

  - Administer Rho(D) immune globulin (RhoGAM) IM around 28 weeks of gestation for clients who are Rh-negative.

- Client education

  - Instruct clients to avoid all over-the-counter medications, supplements, and prescription medications unless prescribed by the provider.

  - Instruct clients to avoid all alcohol, illegal substance and tobacco during pregnancy. Support smoking cessation.

  - Encourage clients to receive a flu vaccine during the fall months.

  - Encourage regular exercise, usually 30 min of moderate exercise (walking or swimming) daily.

  - Instruct clients to avoid the use of hot tubs or saunas.

- Suggest clients consume at least 2 to 3 L of fluid each day from food and beverage sources; preferably milk, water, or juice.

- Show clients how to perform fetal kick counts daily. Fetal activity should be counted two or three times a day for 60 min each time. Fetal movements of less than 3 in/hr or movements that cease entirely for 12 hr indicate a need for further evaluation.

- Provide education about expected psychosocial changes.

- Explain that clients may have unpredictable mood changes and increased irritability, tearfulness, and anger alternating with feelings of joy and cheerfulness. This all may result from dramatic hormonal changes.

  □ Explain that feelings of ambivalence about the pregnancy are a normal response that may occur early in the pregnancy but should resolve before the third trimester. It consists of conflicting feelings (joy, pleasure, sorrow, hostility) about the pregnancy. These feelings can occur simultaneously whether the pregnancy was planned or not.

- Provide education about expected physiological and body image changes.

- Explain that in the first trimester of pregnancy, physiological changes are not very obvious. Many women look forward to the changes so that the pregnancy will be more noticeable.

- Explain that there are rapid physical changes during the second trimester. The most obvious is the enlargement of the abdomen and breasts. Skin changes also occur, such as stretch marks and hyperpigmentation of the face (chloasma). The physical changes can affect mobility and feelings of fatigue, back or leg discomfort and loss of balance may all occur. All of these factors may lead to a negative body image. Clients may make statements of resentment toward the pregnancy and express anxiousness for the pregnancy to be over soon.

- Provide instructions to assist clients with managing common discomforts of pregnancy.

TRIMESTER	DISCOMFORT	CLIENT EDUCATION
First	Nausea and vomiting	• Eat crackers or dry toast 1/2 to 1 hr before rising in the morning. • Drink fluids between meals.
First	Breast tenderness	• Wear a bra that provides adequate support.
First and third	Urinary frequency	• Empty the bladder frequently, decrease fluid intake before bedtime, and use perineal pads. • Perform Kegel exercises (alternate tightening and relaxation of pubococcygeal muscles). Attempt to perform 24 to 100 contractions/day.

TRIMESTER	DISCOMFORT	CLIENT EDUCATION
First, second, third	Urinary tract infections (UTIs)	• Wipe the perineal area from front to back after voiding. Avoid bubble baths and tight-fitting pants. • Wear cotton underpants. • Consume 2 to 3 L of fluid each day from food and beverage sources. • Urinate before and after intercourse to flush bacteria from the urethra. • Urinate as soon as the urge occurs. Notify the provider if urine is malodorous, contains blood or pus, or pain is experienced during urination.
First	Fatigue	• Rest frequently and get adequate sleep at night.
Second, third	Heartburn	• Eat small, frequent meals. • Sit up for 30 min after meals. • Check with the provider prior to using any over-the-counter antacids.
Second, third	Constipation	• Drink plenty of fluids. • Eat a diet high in fiber. • Exercise regularly.
Second, third	Hemorrhoids	• Take warm sitz baths. • Use witch hazel pads and use topical ointments.
Second, third	Backaches	• Exercise regularly. • Perform pelvic tilt exercises (alternately arching and straightening the back). • Use the legs to lift rather than the back. • Use the side-lying position.
Third	Shortness of breath and dyspnea	• Maintain good posture, sleep with extra pillows, and contact the provider if symptoms worsen.
Third	Leg cramps	• Relieve cramps by extending the affected leg, keeping the knee straight and dorsiflexing the foot. • Massage and apply heat over the affected muscle or a foot massage while the leg is extended.

TRIMESTER	DISCOMFORT	CLIENT EDUCATION
Second, third	Varicose veins and lower-extremity edema	• Rest with legs elevated, wear support hose and sleep in the left lateral position. • Avoid constricting clothing, sitting or standing in one position for extended periods of time, and sitting with legs crossed at the knees. • Perform moderate exercise, such as walking.
First	Gingivitis, nasal stuffiness, and epistaxis (nosebleed)	• Use a soft toothbrush and practice good dental hygiene. • Use a humidifier and normal saline nose drops or spray.
Start in first and continue throughout pregnancy	Braxton Hicks contractions	• Change position and walk to decrease discomfort of contractions. • Notify the provider if contractions increase in intensity and frequency (true contractions) with regularity
Second, third	Supine hypotension and bradycardia with feelings of lightheadedness and faintness	• Use a side-lying or semi-sitting position with knees slightly flexed, and change positions slowly.

- Instruct clients to watch for signs of potential complications and to report occurrence to provider.

 View Media Supplement: Danger Signs of Pregnancy (Video)

- Gush of fluid from the vagina (rupture of amniotic membranes) prior to 37 weeks of gestation

- Persistent contractions and abdominal cramping prior to 37 weeks of gestation

- Vaginal bleeding (placental problems such as abruption or previa)

- Abdominal pain (premature labor, abruptio placentae, or ectopic pregnancy)

- Changes in fetal activity (decreased fetal movement may indicate fetal distress)

- Persistent vomiting (hyperemesis gravidarum)

- Severe headaches, blurred vision, edema of face and hands, or epigastric pain (severe preeclampsia))

- Elevated temperature (infection)

- Dysuria (urinary tract infection)

- □ Concurrent occurrence of flushed dry skin, fruity breath, rapid breathing, increased thirst and urination, and headache (hyperglycemia)
- □ Concurrent occurrence of clammy pale skin, weakness, tremors, irritability, and lightheadedness (hypoglycemia)
- Encourage clients to schedule childbirth preparation and/or breastfeeding classes to start during the second or third trimester.
- Discuss options for birth plan and pain management during labor.

(A) APPLICATION EXERCISES

Scenario: A nurse in a provider's office is caring for a client who requested a pregnancy test. She states that her last menstrual period was on April 8. The result of the test is positive. She has been pregnant two other times, delivering a newborn at term who is now 4 years old, and had one miscarriage at 12 weeks.

1. Using Nägele's rule, what is the estimated date of birth (EDB)?

2. Identify the client's obstetrical history using the GTPAL method.

3. The following are presumptive and probable signs of pregnancy. Match each sign nomenclature with its correct explanation.

    _____ Hegar's sign   A. Mask of pregnancy (pigmentation increases on the face)

    _____ Chadwick's sign   B. Slight fluttering movements of fetus felt by the woman

    _____ Goodell's sign   C. Deepened violet-bluish color of vaginal mucosa secondary to increased vascularity of the area

    _____ Ballottement   D. Dark line of pigmentation from the umbilicus to the pubic area

    _____ Braxton Hicks   E. Softening and compressibility of the lower uterus

    _____ Quickening   F. Painless, irregular contractions that are usually relieved with walking

    _____ Chloasma   G. Softening of cervical tip

    _____ Linea nigra   H. Stretch marks most often found on the abdomen and thighs

    _____ Striae gravidarum   I. Rebound of unengaged fetus

4. A nurse is caring for a woman during a prenatal visit. The client is lying supine and suddenly reports feeling breathless. Which of the following findings should the nurse expect if the client is experiencing supine hypotension? (Select all that apply.)

    _____ Dizziness

    _____ Damp, cool skin

    _____ Facial flushing

    _____ Increased heart rate

    _____ Nausea

5. A nurse is planning to obtain initial routine laboratory tests for a pregnant client at 8 weeks of gestation. Which of the following should the nurse anticipate collecting at the prenatal visit?

    A. Beta strep culture

    B. Maternal serum alpha-fetoprotein

    C. One-hour glucose tolerance

    D. Venereal disease research laboratory

6. A nurse is working in a prenatal clinic. When and to whom should the nurse expect to administer Rho(D) immune globulin (RhoGAM) IM?

7. A client who is pregnant should promptly report which of the following symptoms to the provider?

    A. Vaginal bleeding

    B. Swelling of the ankles

    C. Heartburn after eating

    D. Faintness when lying on back

8. A nurse is reinforcing teaching to a group of pregnant women regarding common discomforts during pregnancy. Which of the following occur during the first and third trimesters? (Select all that apply).

    _____ Urinary frequency

    _____ Heartburn

    _____ Dysuria

    _____ Fatigue

    _____ Headaches

(A) APPLICATION EXERCISES ANSWER KEY

Scenario: A nurse in a provider's office is caring for a client who requested a pregnancy test. She states that her last menstrual period was on April 8. The result of the test is positive. She has been pregnant two other times, delivering a newborn at term who is now 4 years old, and had one miscarriage at 12 weeks.

1. Using Nägele's rule, what is the estimated date of birth (EDB)?

   The estimated date of birth is January 15. Nägele's rule can be used to calculate the EDB. Subtracting 3 months from the start of the last menstrual period and adding seven days and one year indicates that her EDB is January 15.

   (N) NCLEX® Connection: Health Promotion and Maintenance, Ante/Intra/Postpartum and Newborn Care

2. Identify the client's obstetrical history using the GTPAL method.

   G 3 T 1 P 0 A 1 L 1; G 3 – The client has been pregnant twice and is currently pregnant; T 1 – the client delivered a newborn at term; P 0 – the client has had no preterm deliveries; A 1 – the client has had one miscarriage; L1– the client has one living child.

   (N) NCLEX® Connection: Health Promotion and Maintenance, Ante/Intra/Postpartum and Newborn Care

3. The following are presumptive and probable signs of pregnancy. Match each sign nomenclature with its correct explanation.

E	Hegar's sign	A. Mask of pregnancy (pigmentation increases on the face)
C	Chadwick's sign	B. Slight fluttering movements of fetus felt by the woman
G	Goodell's sign	C. Deepened violet-bluish color of vaginal mucosa secondary to increased vascularity of the area
I	Ballottement	D. Dark line of pigmentation from the umbilicus to the pubic area
F	Braxton Hicks	E. Softening and compressibility of the lower uterus
B	Quickening	F. Painless, irregular contractions that are usually relieved with walking
A	Chloasma	G. Softening of cervical tip
D	Linea nigra	H. Stretch marks most often found on the abdomen and thighs
H	Striae gravidarum	I. Rebound of unengaged fetus

   (N) NCLEX® Connection: Health Promotion and Maintenance, Ante/Intra/Postpartum and Newborn Care

4. A nurse is caring for a woman during a prenatal visit. The client is lying supine and suddenly reports feeling breathless. Which of the following findings should the nurse expect if the client is experiencing supine hypotension? (Select all that apply.)

    <u>X</u> **Dizziness**

    <u>X</u> **Damp, cool skin**

    _____ Facial flushing

    <u>X</u> **Increased heart rate**

    <u>X</u> **Nausea**

    Signs and symptoms of supine hypotension include dizziness, faintness, damp, cool skin, pallor, tachycardia and nausea. The nurse should encourage the client to use left-lateral positioning to relieve the pressure on the vena cava.

 NCLEX® Connection: Physiological Adaptations, Alterations in Body Systems

5. A nurse is planning to obtain initial routine laboratory tests for a pregnant client at 8 weeks of gestation. Which of the following should the nurse anticipate collecting at the prenatal visit?

    A. Beta strep culture

    B. Maternal serum alpha-fetoprotein

    C. One-hour glucose tolerance

    D. Venereal disease research laboratory

    Venereal disease research laboratory (VDRL) or rapid plasma reagent (RPR) is collected at the initial prenatal visit and mandated by law. The other specimens are obtained for testing as the pregnancy progresses.

 NCLEX® Connection: Health Promotion and Maintenance, Health Promotion/Disease Prevention

6. A nurse is working in a prenatal clinic. When and to whom should the nurse expect to administer Rho(D) immune globulin (RhoGAM) IM?

    Administer Rho(D) immune globulin (RhoGAM) IM around 28 weeks of gestation for clients who are Rh-negative.

 NCLEX® Connection: Pharmacological Therapies, Medication Administration

7. A client who is pregnant should promptly report which of the following symptoms to the provider?

    A. Vaginal bleeding

    B. Swelling of the ankles

    C. Heartburn after eating

    D. Faintness when lying on back

    Vaginal bleeding during pregnancy is always a dangerous sign and the client should notify her provider. Swelling of the ankles is a normal occurrence that can be relieved by the client elevating her lower extremities and not sitting or standing for prolonged periods of time. Heartburn frequently occurs because of the slowed gastrointestinal motility and compression of the stomach by the enlarging uterus. Supine hypotension, which can be experienced by the client as a faintness felt when lying on the back, occurs because of the gravid uterus compressing the ascending vena cava. This compression can be detrimental to the fetus. Supine hypotension is easily rectified by instructing the client to lie on her side or in a semi-sitting position.

    NCLEX® Connection: Health Promotion and Maintenance, Ante/Intra/Postpartum and Newborn Care

8. A nurse is reinforcing teaching to a group of pregnant women regarding common discomforts during pregnancy. Which of the following occur during the first and third trimesters? (Select all that apply).

X	**Urinary frequency**
X	**Heartburn**
	Dysuria
X	**Fatigue**
	Headaches

    Pregnant women commonly report experiencing urinary frequency, heartburn, and fatigue during the first and third trimesters of pregnancy. Headaches and dysuria are danger signs of pregnancy that should be reported to the provider.

    NCLEX® Connection: Health Promotion and Maintenance, Ante/Intra/Postpartum and Newborn Care

UNIT 1	ANTEPARTUM NURSING CARE
Section:	Low-Risk Pregnancy
Chapter 3	Nutrition During Pregnancy

Overview

- Adequate nutritional intake by clients during pregnancy is essential to promoting fetal and maternal health.

- Nurses should use the nursing process to identify potential risk factors, assess current nutritional status, and assist clients to maintain healthy nutritional intake throughout pregnancy and the postpartum period.

- Recommended weight gain during pregnancy is usually 11.2 to 15.9 kg (25 to 35 lb). The general rule is that clients should gain 1 to 2 kg (3 to 4 lb) during the first trimester and after that, a weight gain of approximately 0.4 kg (1 lb) per week for the last two trimesters. The provider may recommend more or less based on the client's current weight or body mass index (BMI).

Risk Factors

- Adolescence

  o Lack of information

  o Poor adherence to prescribed supplements

  o Dietary intake may be inadequate to meet the nutritional needs of the mother and the fetus (low intake of protein and vitamins)

  o Nutritional habits may include erratic eating schedule, high intake of processed foods, and beverages high in sugar content and caffeine

  o The equivalent of 500 to 750 mL/day of coffee may increase the risk of a spontaneous abortion or fetal intrauterine growth restriction.

- Specific diets

  o Vegetarian diet may be low in protein, calcium, iron, zinc, and vitamin

- Medical disorders

  o Hyperemesis gravidarum

  o Anemia

  o Eating disorders such as anorexia nervosa or bulimia

- ○ Pica – Craving to eat nonfood substances such as dirt or red clay. This disorder may interfere with adequate nutritional intake.

- ○ Excessive weight gain can lead to macrosomia and labor complications.

- ○ Inability to gain weight may result in low birth weight of the newborn.

- ○ Financially unable to purchase/access food.

Data Collection

- Subjective and objective data

  - ○ Daily food intake to include amount of protein, calcium and folic acid

  - ○ Food intolerances

  - ○ Caffeine and alcohol consumption

  - ○ Baseline height and weight

  - ○ Laboratory reports such as Hgb and iron levels

Nursing Interventions

- Monitor weight at each prenatal visit.

- Reinforce the following guidelines during pregnancy:

  - ○ Increase daily calories by 340 calories/day during the second trimester.

  - ○ Increase daily calories by 452 calories/day during the third trimester.

  - ○ Increase protein intake from 46 g to 71 g during pregnancy.

  - ○ Consume 600 mcg of folic acid/day. Foods high in folic acid include leafy vegetables, dried peas and beans, seeds, and orange juice. Breads, cereals, and other grains are fortified with folic acid (Folic acid supplements are recommended for all women of childbearing age).

  - ○ Take iron supplements as prescribed. Take between meals and with a good source of vitamin C; avoid milk and caffeine intake at the same time.

  - ○ Eat a diet that includes good sources of iron such as beef liver, red meats, fish, poultry, dried peas and beans, and fortified cereals and breads. Take an OTC stool softener if constipation occurs.

  - ○ Consume an adequate amount of calcium from food sources such as calcium-fortified soy milk and orange juice, nuts, legumes, and dark green leafy vegetables. Daily recommendation is 1,000 mg/day for pregnant women over the age of 19, and 1,300 mg/day for those under 19 years of age.

  - ○ Consume 2 to 3 L of fluids from food and beverage sources daily. Fluids that are preferable include water, fruit juice, or milk.

  - ○ Limit caffeine intake to 300 mg/day.

  - ○ Abstain from all alcohol consumption.

- o Obtain weight at each prenatal visit. Monitor for appropriate weight gain.

- o Provide written materials regarding nutrition.

- o Identify the need for community resources. Assist clients to obtain access to necessary resources. Woman Infants and Children (WIC) is a federally funded program that offers assistance with food available for pregnant women and their children (up to 5 years old).

- Instruct clients to adhere to the following guidelines during the postpartum period.

  - o For lactation

    - Increase daily caloric intake by 330 calories/day during the first 6 months.

    - Increase daily caloric intake to 400 calories/day during the second 6 months.

    - Consume 500 mcg of folic acid.

    - Continue to consume 2 to 3 L of fluids. Drink a glass of fluid each time the infant breastfeeds.

    - Continue to consume 71 g of protein and 1,000 mg of calcium.

    - Avoid alcohol and limit caffeine intake.

    - Avoid food substances that do not agree with the newborn (foods that may cause increased gas).

    - Adhere to a recommended, well-balanced diet.

  - o For nonlactating mothers

    - Adhere to a recommended, well-balanced diet.

Complications

- Nausea

  - o Nursing actions

    - Monitor clients for fluid and electrolyte imbalances.

  - o Client education

    - Tell clients to eat dry crackers or toast.

    - Encourage clients to avoid alcohol, caffeine, fats, and spices.

    - Avoid drinking fluids with meals.

    - Remind clients not to take any medications to control nausea without first checking with the provider.

    - Eat small, frequent meals.

- Constipation
  - Client education
    - Suggest that clients maintain adequate fluid intake and consume food high in fiber (raw fruits and vegetables and whole grains).
- Maternal phenylketonuria (PKU) – This is a maternal genetic disease in which high levels of phenylalanine pose danger to the fetus.
  - Nursing actions
    - Monitor the client's blood phenylalanine levels during pregnancy.
  - Client education
    - Instruct clients to consume a diet low in phenylalanine for at least 3 months prior to pregnancy and to continue the diet throughout pregnancy. The diet should include foods that are low in phenylalanine. Foods high in protein, such as fish, poultry, meat, eggs, nuts, and dairy products, must be avoided due to high phenylalanine levels.

Ⓐ APPLICATION EXERCISES

1. A nurse working in a prenatal clinic is providing education to a client who is pregnant. The client does not like milk. Which of the following is a good source of calcium that the nurse can recommend to the client?

    A. Artichokes

    B. Sweet potatoes

    C. Apricots

    D. Turnip greens

2. A nurse is reinforcing nutritional education to a client. Which of the following statements made by the client indicate a need for further teaching?

    A. "I will drink 2 to 3 liters of fluid daily."

    B. "It is important to consume 600 mcg of folic acid each day."

    C. "I should eat an additional 300 calories per day in my third trimester."

    D. "My protein intake should be around 50 g each day during my pregnancy."

3. A nurse is reinforcing teaching with a pregnant client who is diagnosed with iron deficiency anemia and has been prescribed iron supplements. Which of the following statements made by the client indicates an understanding of the teaching?

    A. "I will take the iron with ice water."

    B. "I will drink low-fat or whole milk with my iron."

    C. "I should drink tea or coffee with my medication."

    D. "I should take the medication with orange juice."

APPLICATION EXERCISES ANSWER KEY

1. A nurse working in a prenatal clinic is providing education to a client who is pregnant. The client does not like milk. Which of the following is a good source of calcium that the nurse can recommend to the client?

   A. Artichokes

   B. Sweet potatoes

   C. Apricots

   D. Turnip greens

   Calcium is very important to a developing fetus. It is involved in bone and teeth formation. Good sources of calcium include calcium-fortified orange juice, nuts, legumes, and low-oxalate, dark green, leafy vegetables. Sweet potatoes, artichokes, and apricots are rich in potassium.

   Ⓝ NCLEX® Connection: Health Promotion and Maintenance, Ante/Intra/Postpartum and Newborn Care

2. A nurse is reinforcing nutritional education to a client. Which of the following statements made by the client indicate a need for further teaching?

   A. "I will drink 2 to 3 liters of fluid daily."

   B. "It is important to consume 600 mcg of folic acid each day."

   C. "I should eat an additional 300 calories per day in my third trimester."

   D. "My protein intake should be around 50 g each day during my pregnancy."

   Caloric needs increase during the third trimester by 452 calories/day. Therefore, this statement requires additional teaching. Pregnant clients should drink 2 to 3 L of fluid and consume 600 mcg of folic acid and 46 to 71 g of protein daily.

   Ⓝ NCLEX® Connection: Health Promotion and Maintenance, Ante/Intra/Postpartum and Newborn Care

3. A nurse is reinforcing teaching with a pregnant client who is diagnosed with iron deficiency anemia and has been prescribed iron supplements. Which of the following statements made by the client indicates an understanding of the teaching?

   A. "I will take the iron with ice water."

   B. "I will drink low-fat or whole milk with my iron."

   C. "I should drink tea or coffee with my medication."

   D. "I should take the medication with orange juice."

   Orange juice contains vitamin C, which aids in the absorption of iron. Milk and caffeine interfere with iron absorption. Also, caffeine intake from tea and coffee should be limited to 300 mg daily because caffeine increases the risk of a spontaneous abortion or fetal intrauterine growth restriction. Water will not help with the absorption of iron.

   Ⓝ NCLEX® Connection: Health Promotion and Maintenance: Ante/ Intra/ Postpartum and Newborn Care

UNIT 1	ANTEPARTUM NURSING CARE
Section:	Low-Risk Pregnancy
Chapter 4	Assessment of Fetal Well-Being

Overview

- Various diagnostic tests may be used to determine the well-being of a fetus during pregnancy.

- These diagnostic procedures include ultrasound (abdominal, transvaginal, Doppler), biophysical profile, nonstress test, contraction stress test (nipple, oxytocin [Pitocin]), amniocentesis, percutaneous umbilical cord blood sampling, chorionic villus sampling, quad marker screening, and maternal serum alpha-fetoprotein.

ULTRASONOGRAPHY (ABDOMINAL, TRANSVAGINAL, DOPPLER)

Overview

- Ultrasonography – A procedure lasting approximately 20 min that consists of high-frequency sound waves used to visualize internal organs and tissues by producing a real-time, three-dimensional pictorial image of the developing fetus and maternal structures (FHR, pelvic anatomy). An ultrasound allows for an early diagnosis of complications, permitting earlier interventions, and thereby decreasing the neonate's and mother's morbidity and mortality.

  o External abdominal ultrasonography – A noninvasive, painless, and safe procedure. Ultrasonic/transducer gel, that is warmed or is at room temperature, is applied to the client's abdomen and then the ultrasound transducer is moved over the abdomen to obtain an image.

  o Internal transvaginal ultrasonography – An invasive procedure in which a vaginal probe covered with a condom and lubricated with ultrasonic gel is inserted vaginally to allow for a more accurate evaluation. It is useful in the first trimester to detect an ectopic pregnancy, identify abnormalities, and to establish gestational age.

  o Doppler blood flow analysis – An external ultrasonography method of noninvasively studying the maternal-fetal blood flow. It is useful in fetal intrauterine growth restriction (IUGR), identifying poor placental perfusion, and as an adjunct in pregnancies at risk because of hypertension, diabetes mellitus, multiple fetuses, or preterm labor.

- Indications
  - Confirm pregnancy, number of fetuses, and gestational age.
  - Assess fetal growth and development.
  - Confirm fetal viability or death (Reports of decreased fetal movement).
  - Rule out or verify fetal abnormalities.
  - Locate the site of placental attachment.
  - Determine amniotic fluid volume.
  - Observe for fetal movement (fetal heartbeat, breathing, and activity).
  - Adjunct for other procedures (amniocentesis, biophysical profile).
- Interpretation of Findings
  - Confirm pregnancy, number of fetuses, and gestational age.
  - Appropriate growth and development or intrauterine growth restriction.
- Preprocedure
  - Nursing actions
    - Assist the client into a supine position with a wedge placed under the right hip to displace the uterus (prevent supine hypotension).
    - For pregnancies less than 12 weeks of gestation, the client may be asked to have a full bladder for an abdominal ultrasound.
    - For a transvaginal ultrasound:
      - Ask the client to undress from the waist down.
      - Assist the client into the supine position with the legs in stirrups.
      - Drape the client appropriately.
    - Client education
      - Explain the procedure to the client and reinforce that it presents no known risk to her or her fetus.
      - Inform the client that results will usually not be given by the provider at the time of the procedure, but at a later date.
      - Advise the client to drink 1 to 2 q of fluid prior to the procedure; if indicated.
- Intraprocedure
  - Nursing actions
    - Monitor the client for supine hypotension.

- Postprocedure

  - Nursing actions

    - Allow the client to empty the bladder at the termination of the procedure.

BIOPHYSICAL PROFILE

Overview

- Biophysical profile (BPP) – Uses a real-time ultrasound to visualize physical and physiological characteristics of the fetus and observes for fetal biophysical responses to stimuli.

- BPP assesses the fetal well-being by measuring the following five variables with a score of 2 for each normal finding, and 0 for each abnormal finding for each variable.

  - Reactive FHR (reactive nonstress test [NST]) = 2; nonreactive NST = 0.

  - Fetal breathing movements (at least 1 episode of 30 sec in 30 min) = 2; absent or less than 30 sec duration = 0.

  - Gross body movements (at least 3 body or limb extensions with return to flexion in 30 min) = 2; less than 3 episodes = 0.

  - Fetal tone (at least 1 episode of extension with return to flexion) = 2; slow extension and flexion, lack of flexion, or absent of movement = 0.

  - Amniotic fluid volume (at least 1 pocket of fluid that measures at least 1 cm in two perpendicular planes) = 2; pockets absent or less than 1 cm = 0.

- Indications

  - Potential diagnoses

    - Suspected oligohydramnios or polyhydramnios

    - Suspected fetal hypoxemia and/or hypoxia

- Client Presentation

  - Premature rupture of membranes

  - Maternal infection

  - Decreased fetal movement

  - NST or contraction stress test

  - Intrauterine growth restriction

- Interpretation of Findings

  - Total score of 8 to 10 is normal

  - 6 is equivocal

  - Less than 4 is abnormal

- Preprocedure

  o Nursing actions

    ▪ Follow the same nursing actions as those used for an ultrasound.

NONSTRESS TEST (NST)

 Overview

- Nonstress test (NST) – A noninvasive procedure that monitors response of the FHR to fetal movement. A Doppler transducer, used to monitor the FHR, and a tocotransducer, used to monitor uterine contractions, is attached externally to a client's abdomen to obtain a tracing. The client pushes a button attached to the monitor whenever she feels a fetal movement, which is then noted on the tracing. This allows a nurse to assess the FHR in relationship to the fetal movement.

  o NSTs include a high rate of false nonreactive results with the fetal movement response affected by sleep cycles of the fetus, fetal immaturity, maternal medications, and chronic smoking.

- Indications

  o Client presentation

    ▪ Decreased fetal movement

    ▪ Intrauterine growth restriction

    ▪ Postmaturity

    ▪ Gestational diabetes mellitus

    ▪ Preeclampsia

    ▪ Maternal chronic hypertension

    ▪ History of previous fetal demise

    ▪ Advanced maternal age

    ▪ Sickle cell disease

- Interpretation of Findings

  o The NST is interpreted as reactive if the FHR is normal baseline rate with moderate variability, FHR accelerates to 15/min for at least 15 seconds and occurs two or more times during a 20-min period.

  View Media Supplement: Reactive NST (Image)

  o A nonreactive NST indicates that the fetal heart rate does not accelerate adequately with fetal movement and does not meet the above criteria after 40 min. Additional assessment is indicated, such as a CST or biophysical profile (BPP).

- Nursing Actions

    o Preparation of the client

        ▪ Seat the client in a reclining chair or place in a semi-Fowler's or left-lateral position.

        ▪ Perform Leopold's maneuvers to locate the fetal back.

        ▪ Apply conduction gel to the ultrasound transducer.

        ▪ Secure a Doppler transducer on the client's abdomen over the fetal back to record the FHR pattern. A tocodynamometer should be secured over the fundus to record the uterine contractions.

    o Ongoing care

        ▪ Instruct the client to press the button on the handheld event marker each time she feels the fetus move.

        ▪ If there are no fetal movements (fetus sleeping), vibroacoustic stimulation (sound source, usually laryngeal stimulator) may be activated for 3 seconds on the maternal abdomen over the fetal head to awaken a sleeping fetus.

        ▪ If NST is still nonreactive, anticipate a CST and/or BPP.

CONTRACTION STRESS TEST (CST)

Overview

- A nipple stimulated CST is performed by the client by lightly brushing her palm across her nipple for 2 or 3 min, which causes the pituitary gland to release endogenous oxytocin, and then stopping the nipple stimulation when a contraction begins. The same process is repeated after a 5 min rest period.

    o This should stimulate contractions (which decrease placental blood flow) and then the FHR is analyzed in conjunction with the contractions to determine how the fetus will tolerate the stress of labor. A pattern of at least three contractions within a 10- min time period with duration of 40 to 60 seconds each must be obtained to use for assessment data.

    o Avoid hyperstimulation of the uterus (uterine contraction longer than 90 seconds or more frequent than every 2 min) by stimulating the nipple intermittently with rest periods in between, and avoiding bimanual stimulation of both nipples unless stimulation of one nipple is unsuccessful.

- Oxytocin (Pitocin) administration CST is used if nipple stimulation fails and involves the IV administration of oxytocin to induce uterine contractions.

    o Contractions started with oxytocin may be difficult to stop and can lead to preterm labor

- Indications

  - Potential diagnoses

    - High-risk pregnancies (gestational diabetes mellitus, postterm pregnancy).

  - Client presentation

    - Decreased fetal movement

    - Nonreactive NST

    - Intrauterine growth restriction

    - Postmaturity

    - Gestational diabetes mellitus

    - Gestational hypertension

    - Preeclampsia

    - Maternal chronic hypertension

    - History of previous fetal demise

    - Advanced maternal age

    - Sickle-cell disease

- Interpretation of Findings

  - A negative CST (normal finding) is indicated if within a 10-min period, with three uterine contractions, there are no late decelerations of the FHR.

  - A positive CST (abnormal finding) is determined when persistent and consistent late decelerations are present with more than half of the contractions. This is suggestive of uteroplacental insufficiency. Variable deceleration may indicate cord compression, and early decelerations may indicate fetal head compression. Based on these findings, the primary care provider may determine to induce labor or perform a cesarean birth.

- Preprocedure

  - Nursing actions

    - Obtain a baseline FHR, fetal movement, and contractions for 10 to 20 min and document.

  - Client education

    - Explain the procedure to the client and ensure that an informed consent form has been signed.

- Intraprocedure

  - Nursing actions

    - Initiate nipple stimulation if there are no contractions. Instruct the client to roll a nipple between her thumb and fingers or brush her palm across her nipple. The client should stop when a uterine contraction begins.

- - Monitor and provide adequate rest periods for the client to avoid hyperstimulation of the uterus.

    - Assist with monitoring the client receiving IV oxytocin.

    - Monitor for contractions lasting longer than 90 seconds and/or occurring more frequently than every 2 min.

        □ Maintain bed rest during the procedure.

- Postprocedure

    o Nursing actions

        - Observe the client for 30 min afterward to see that contractions have ceased and preterm labor does not begin.

- Complications

    o Potential for preterm labor

AMNIOCENTESIS

 Overview

- Amniocentesis – The aspiration of amniotic fluid for analysis by insertion of a needle transabdominally into a client's uterus and amniotic sac under direct ultrasound guidance locating the placenta and determining the position of the fetus. It may be performed after 14 weeks of gestation.

- Indications

    o Potential diagnoses

        - Maternal age greater than 35 years

        - Previous birth with a chromosomal anomaly

        - A parent who is a carrier of a chromosomal anomaly

        - A family history of neural tube defects

        - Lung maturity assessment

        - Fetal hemolytic disease diagnosis

- Interpretation of Findings

    o Alpha-fetoprotein (AFP) can be measured from the amniotic fluid between 16 and 18 weeks of gestation and may be used to assess for neural tube defects in the fetus or chromosomal disorders. May be evaluated to follow up a high level of AFP in maternal serum.

        - High levels of AFP are associated with neural tube defects such as anencephaly (incomplete development of fetal skull and brain), spina bifida (open spine), or omphalocele (abdominal wall defect). High AFP levels may also be present with normal multifetal pregnancies.

- Low levels of AFP are associated with chromosomal disorders (Down syndrome) or gestational trophoblastic disease (hydatidiform mole).

  ○ Tests for fetal lung maturity may be performed if gestation is less than 37 weeks, in the event of a rupture of membranes, for preterm labor, or for a complication indicating a cesarean birth. Amniotic fluid is tested to determine if the fetal lungs are mature enough to adapt to extrauterine life or if the fetus will likely have respiratory distress.

    - Fetal lung tests

      □ Lecithin/sphingomyelin (L/S) ratio – A 2:1 indicating fetal lung maturity (2.5:1 or 3:1 for a client who has diabetes mellitus).

      □ Presence of phosphatidylglycerol (PG) – Absence of PG is associated with respiratory distress

- Preprocedure

  ○ Nursing actions

    - Explain the procedure to the client and ensure an informed consent form has been signed.

  ○ Client education

    - Instruct the client to empty her bladder prior to the procedure.

- Intraprocedure

  ○ Nursing actions

    - Assist the client into a supine position and place a wedge or rolled towel under her right hip to displace the uterus off the vena cava and place a drape over the client exposing only her abdomen.

    - Prepare the client for an ultrasound to locate the placenta.

    - Obtain the client's baseline vital signs and FHR and document prior to the procedure.

    - Cleanse the client's abdomen with an antiseptic solution prior to the administration of a local anesthetic given by the provider.

  ○ Client education

    - Advise the client that she will feel slight pressure as the needle is inserted for aspiration.

- Postprocedure

  ○ Nursing actions

    - Monitor the client's vital signs, FHR, and uterine contractions throughout and 30 min following the procedure.

    - Have the client rest for 30 min.

    - Administer Rho(D) immune globulin (RhoGAM) to the client if she is Rh-negative.

- ○ Client education
  - Encourage the client to drink plenty of liquids and rest for the next 24 hr postprocedure.
- ○ Complications
  - Amniotic fluid emboli
  - Maternal or fetal hemorrhage
  - Fetomaternal hemorrhage with Rh isoimmunization
  - Maternal or fetal infection
  - Inadvertent fetal damage or anomalies involving limbs
  - Fetal death
  - Inadvertent maternal intestinal or bladder damage
  - Miscarriage or preterm labor
  - Premature rupture of membranes
  - Leakage of amniotic fluid
- ○ Nursing actions
  - Monitor the client's vital signs, temperature, respiratory status, FHR, uterine contractions, and vaginal discharge for amniotic fluid or bleeding.
- ○ Client education
  - Advise the client to notify the provider if she experiences fever, chills, leakage of fluid, or bleeding from the insertion site, decreased fetal movement, vaginal bleeding, or uterine contractions after the procedure.

PERCUTANEOUS UMBILICAL BLOOD SAMPLING (PUBS)

Overview

- Percutaneous umbilical blood sampling (PUBS) – the most common method used for sampling fetal blood. This procedure obtains fetal blood sampling from the umbilical cord by passing a fine-gauge fiber optic scope (fetoscope) into the amniotic sac using the amniocentesis technique. The needle is advanced into the umbilical cord under ultrasound guidance and blood is aspirated from the umbilical vein. Blood studies from the cordocentesis may consist of:
  - ○ Kleihauer-Betke test that ensures blood obtained is from the fetus.
  - ○ CBC count with differential.
  - ○ Indirect Coombs' test for Rh antibodies.
  - ○ Karyotyping (visualization of chromosomes).
  - ○ Blood gases.

- Indications
    - Potential diagnoses
        - Diagnosing prenatal blood and chromosomal disorders
        - Karyotyping of malformed fetuses
        - Detecting of fetal infection
        - Determining the acid-base balance status of fetuses with IUGR
- Interpretation of Findings
    - Evaluate for isoimmune fetal hemolytic anemia and assessing the need for a fetal blood transfusion.
- Complications
    - Cord laceration
    - Preterm labor
    - Amnionitis

CHORIONIC VILLUS SAMPLING (CVS)

Overview

- Chorionic villus sampling (CVS) – Assessment of a portion of the developing placenta (chorionic villi) that is aspirated through a thin sterile catheter or syringe through the abdomen or intravaginally through the cervix under ultrasound guidance.
    - CVS is a first-trimester alternative to amniocentesis, with one of its advantages being an earlier diagnosis of any abnormalities. CVS can be performed at 10 to 12 weeks of gestation and rapid results with chromosome studies are available in 24 to 48 hr following aspiration.
- Indications
    - Potential diagnoses
        - Women at risk for giving birth to a newborn who has a genetic chromosomal abnormality (cannot determine spina bifida or anencephaly)
    - Client education
        - Provide ongoing education and support.
        - Instruct the client to drink plenty of fluid to fill the bladder prior to the procedure to assist in positioning the uterus for catheter insertion.
- Complications
    - Spontaneous abortion (higher risk with CVS than with amniocentesis)
    - Risk for fetal limb loss

- o   Miscarriage

- o   Chorioamnionitis and rupture of membranes

QUAD MARKER AND ALPHA-FETOPROTEIN (MSAFP) SCREENING

Overview

- Quad Marker screening – A blood test done between 15 to 20 weeks of gestation that will ascertain information about the likelihood of fetal birth defects. It does not diagnose the actual defect. It may be performed instead of the maternal serum alpha-fetoprotein yielding more reliable findings. The test screens for the presence of hCG, AFP, estriol and Inhibin-A.

  - o   Human chorionic gonadotropin (hCG) – A hormone produced by the placenta

  - o   Alpha-fetoprotein (AFP) – A protein produced by the fetus

  - o   Estriol – A protein produced by the fetus and placenta

  - o   Inhibin-A – A protein produced by the ovaries and placenta

- Indications

  - o   Client presentation

    - ▪   15 to 20 weeks gestation

    - ▪   Women at risk for giving birth to a newborn who has a genetic chromosomal abnormality

- Interpretation of Findings

  - o   Low levels of AFP may indicate a risk for Down syndrome.

  - o   High levels of AFP may indicate a risk for neural tube defects.

  - o   Higher levels than normal of hCG and Inhibin-A indicates a risk for Down syndrome.

  - o   Lower levels than normal of estriol may indicate a risk for Down syndrome.

- Description of Procedure

  - o   Maternal serum AFP is a screening tool used to detect neural tube defects. Clients with abnormal findings should be referred for a quad marker screening, genetic counseling, ultrasound, and an amniocentesis.

- Indications

  - o   Potential diagnoses

    - ▪   All pregnant clients between 16 to 18 weeks of gestation

- Interpretation of Findings

  - o   High levels may indicate a neural tube defect or open abdominal defect.

  - o   Lower levels may indicate Down syndrome.

- Preprocedure
  - Nursing actions
    - Discuss testing with the client.
    - Draw blood sample.
  - Client education
    - Provide support and education as needed.

(A) APPLICATION EXERCISES

1. A nurse is aware that a Doppler ultrasound blood flow analysis is useful in which of the following situations? (Select all that apply.)

   _____ Intrauterine growth restriction

   _____ Maternal hypertension

   _____ Poor placenta perfusion

   _____ Hyperemesis gravidarum

   _____ Multiple fetuses

2. A nurse in an antepartum clinic is reviewing the medical record of a client who is in preterm labor and has undergone an amniocentesis. She also had fetal lung maturity testing to determine if her fetus will develop respiratory distress. Which of the following is a test for fetal lung maturity?

   A. Alpha fetoprotein

   B. Lecithin/sphingomyelin ratio

   C. Kleihauer-Betke test

   D. Indirect Coombs' test

3. A nurse determines that a client who is pregnant needs further instructions about an amniocentesis when the client states:

   A. "I must report cramping or signs of infection to the physician."

   B. "I should drink lots of fluids for the next 24 hr following the procedure."

   C. "I need to have a full bladder for the procedure to be done."

   D. "I know that the amniotic fluid can be tested to detect for genetic abnormalities."

4. A nurse is aware that an ultrasound may be prescribed for which of the following indications? (Select all that apply.)

   _____ Questionable rupture of membranes

   _____ Vaginal bleeding

   _____ Uterine contractions

   _____ Preterm labor

   _____ Decreased fetal movement

5. Which of the following findings from a client who is pregnant should indicate to the nurse that the client should undergo an amniocentesis? (Select all that apply.)

   _____ Maternal age greater than 35 years old

   _____ Previous birth with a chromosomal anomaly

   _____ A family history of neural tube defects

   _____ Lung maturity assessment

   _____ Abruptio placentae

6. Explain how to interpret a reactive nonstress test.

(A) **APPLICATION EXERCISES ANSWER KEY**

1. A nurse is aware that a Doppler ultrasound blood flow analysis is useful in which of the following situations? (Select all that apply.)

   __X__ **Intrauterine growth restriction**

   __X__ **Maternal hypertension**

   __X__ **Poor placenta perfusion**

   _____ Hyperemesis gravidarum

   __X__ **Multiple fetuses**

   A Doppler ultrasound blood flow analysis is a noninvasive external ultrasound method of studying the maternal-fetal blood flow. It is especially useful in fetal intrauterine growth restriction (IUGR), identifying poor placental perfusion, and as an adjunct in pregnancies at risk because of multiple fetuses, preterm labor, maternal hypertension, or diabetes mellitus. This tool assists in determining fetal well-being. It is not an assessment tool used for clients with hyperemesis gravidarum.

   (N) NCLEX® Connection: Reduction of Risk Potential, Diagnostic Tests

2. A nurse in an antepartum clinic is reviewing the medical record of a client who is in preterm labor and has undergone an amniocentesis. She also had fetal lung maturity testing to determine if her fetus will develop respiratory distress. Which of the following is a test for fetal lung maturity?

   A. Alpha fetoprotein

   B. Lecithin/sphingomyelin ratio

   C. Kleihauer-Betke test

   D. Indirect Coombs' test

   Lecithin/sphingomyelin (L/S) ratio of 2 to 1 indicates fetal lung maturity (3 to 1 for clients who have diabetes mellitus). Alpha-fetoprotein (AFP) can be measured from the maternal serum between 16 and 18 weeks gestation and may be used to assess for neural tube defects in the fetus or chromosomal disorders. The Kleihauer-Betke test is used to ensure blood is obtained from the fetus during PUBS. The indirect Coombs' test is used to detect Rh antibodies in the mother's blood.

   (N) NCLEX® Connection: Reduction of Risk Potential, Diagnostic Tests

3. A nurse determines that a client who is pregnant needs further instructions about an amniocentesis when the client states:

    A. "I must report cramping or signs of infection to the physician."

    B. "I should drink lots of fluids for the next 24 hr following the procedure."

    C. "I need to have a full bladder for the procedure to be done."

    D. "I know that the amniotic fluid can be tested to detect for genetic abnormalities."

    A full bladder may be necessary for an abdominal ultrasound and chorionic villus sampling. Amniocentesis requires an empty bladder to prevent an inadvertent puncture from occurring. The client should report any signs of infection to the primary care provider and should drink plenty of fluids and rest for 24 hr following the procedure. The amniocentesis is used to detect genetic abnormalities.

 NCLEX® Connection: Reduction of Risk Potential, Diagnostic Tests

4. A nurse is aware that an ultrasound may be prescribed for which of the following indications? (Select all that apply.)

__X__	**Questionable rupture of membranes**
__X__	**Vaginal bleeding**
_____	Uterine contractions
__X__	**Preterm labor**
__X__	**Decreased fetal movement**

    An ultrasound is prescribed for clients who present with vaginal bleeding, preterm labor, decreased fetal movement, and questionable rupture of membranes. Uterine contractions are not an indication for an ultrasound.

 NCLEX® Connection: Reduction of Risk Potential, Diagnostic Tests

5. Which of the following findings from a client who is pregnant should indicate to the nurse that the client should undergo an amniocentesis? (Select all that apply.)

__X__	**Maternal age greater than 35 years old**
__X__	**Previous birth with a chromosomal anomaly**
__X__	**A family history of neural tube defects**
__X__	**Lung maturity assessment**
_____	Abruptio placentae

    Maternal age greater than 35 years old, previous birth with a chromosomal anomaly, familiar history of neural tube defects, and assessment of fetal lung maturity are all indications for an amniocentesis. Abruptio placentae is not an indication for an amniocentesis.

 NCLEX® Connection: Reduction of Risk Potential, Diagnostic Tests

6. Explain how to interpret a reactive nonstress test.

   The FHR accelerates to 15/min for at least 15 seconds and occurs two or more times during a 20 min period.

 NCLEX® Connection: Reduction of Risk Potential, Diagnostic Tests

UNIT 1	ANTEPARTUM NURSING CARE
Section:	Complications of Pregnancy
Chapter 5	Bleeding During Pregnancy

◎ Overview

- Vaginal bleeding during pregnancy is always abnormal and must be investigated to determine the cause. It can impair both the outcome of the pregnancy and the mother's life.

BLEEDING DURING PREGNANCY		
TIME	COMPLICATION	SIGNS AND SYMPTOMS
First trimester	Spontaneous abortion	Vaginal bleeding, uterine cramping, and partial or complete expulsion of products of conception
	Ectopic pregnancy	Abrupt unilateral lower-quadrant abdominal pain with or without vaginal bleeding
Second trimester	Gestational trophoblastic disease	Uterine size increasing abnormally fast, abnormally high levels of hCG, nausea and increased emesis, no fetus present on ultrasound, and scant or profuse dark brown or red vaginal bleeding
Third trimester	Placenta previa	Painless vaginal bleeding
	Abruptio placentae	Vaginal bleeding, sharp abdominal pain, and tender rigid uterus
	Vasa previa	Fetal vessels cross over the cervix, abrupt bright red vaginal bleeding following rupture of membranes

- Other Causes of Bleeding
  - Incompetent cervix
    - Painless bleeding with cervical dilation leading to fetal expulsion
  - Preterm labor
    - Pink-stained vaginal discharge, uterine contractions becoming regular, cervical dilation and effacement

SPONTANEOUS ABORTION

Overview

- Spontaneous abortion occurs when a pregnancy is terminated before 20 weeks of gestation (the point of fetal viability) or a fetal weight less than 500 g.

- Types of abortion are clinically classified according to symptoms and whether the products of conception are partially or completely retained or expulsed. Types of spontaneous abortions include threatened, inevitable, incomplete, complete, missed, septic, and recurrent.

Data Collection

- Risk Factors

  o Chromosomal abnormalities (account for 50%)

  o Maternal illness, such as insulin-dependent diabetes mellitus

  o Advancing maternal age

  o Premature cervical dilation

  o Chronic maternal infections

  o Maternal malnutrition

  o Trauma or injury

  o Fetal or placental anomalies

  o Substance abuse

- Subjective and Objective Data

  o Backache

  o Rupture of membranes

  o Dilation of the cervix

  o Fever

  o Abdominal tenderness

  o Clinical manifestations of hemorrhage such as hypotension and tachycardia

TYPE	CRAMPS	BLEEDING	TISSUE PASSED	CERVICAL OPENING
Threatened	With or without slight cramps	Spotting to moderate	None	Closed

TYPE	CRAMPS	BLEEDING	TISSUE PASSED	CERVICAL OPENING
Inevitable	Moderate	Mild to severe	None	Dilated with membranes or tissues bulging at cervix
Incomplete	Severe	Continuous and severe	Partial fetal tissue or placenta	Dilated with tissue in cervical canal or passage of tissue
Complete	Mild	Minimal	Complete expulsion of uterine contents	Closed with no tissue in cervical canal
Missed	None	Brownish discharge	None, prolonged retention of tissue	Closed
Septic	Mild	Malodorous discharge	Varies	Usually dilated
Recurrent	Varies	Varies	Yes	Usually dilated

- ○ Laboratory tests
    - ▪ Hgb and Hct, if considerable blood loss
    - ▪ Clotting factors monitored for disseminated intravascular coagulopathy (DIC) – a complication with retained products of conception
    - ▪ WBC for suspected infection
    - ▪ Serum human chorionic gonadotropin (hCG) levels to confirm pregnancy
- ○ Diagnostic procedures
    - ▪ An ultrasound is used to determine the presence or absence of fetal well-being, or partial or complete products of conception within the uterine cavity.
    - ▪ An examination of the cervix to determine if it is opened or closed.

Collaborative Care

- • Nursing Care
    - ○ Monitor the amount and color of vaginal bleeding (counting pads).
    - ○ Perform a pregnancy test.
    - ○ Use the lay term "miscarriage" with clients, because "abortion" will likely sound insensitive.

- o Maintain clients on bed rest and administer sedation as prescribed for threatened, inevitable, and incomplete abortions.

- o Avoid performing a vaginal exam.

- o Assist with an ultrasound.

- o Administer analgesics as prescribed.

- o Monitor clients receiving blood transfusions.

- o Provide client education and emotional support.

- Medications

  - o Rho(D) immune globulin (RhoGAM)

  - o Suppresses the immune response of clients who are Rh-negative to Rh-positive RBCs from the fetus.

  - o Nursing considerations

    - Administer Rho(D) immune globulin to clients who are Rh-negative.

    - Administer broad-spectrum antibiotics for treatment of septic abortion.

    - Assist with the care of clients who are receiving prostaglandins or oxytocin (Pitocin) to expulse products of conception in late, incomplete, inevitable, or missed abortions.

- Therapeutic procedures

  - o Dilation and curettage (D&C) is done to dilate and scrape the uterine walls to remove uterine contents for inevitable and incomplete abortions.

  - o Dilation and evacuation (D&E) is done to remove uterine contents after 16 weeks of gestation.

- Care After Discharge

  - o Client education

    - Instruct clients to notify the provider of heavy, bright red vaginal bleeding.

    - Instruct clients to complete course of prescribed antibiotics.

    - Tell clients that a small amount of discharge is normal for 1 to 2 weeks.

    - Instruct clients to refrain from sexual intercourse or placing anything into the vagina for 2 weeks.

    - Provide contacts for bereavement support groups.

    - Instruct clients to avoid pregnancy for 2 months.

- Client Outcomes

  - o The client will experience no physiological complications.

  - o The client will have adequate psychological support to deal with the loss effectively.

ECTOPIC PREGNANCY

Overview

- Ectopic pregnancy is the abnormal implantation of a fertilized ovum outside of the uterine cavity. The implantation is usually in the fallopian tube, which can result in a rupture of the fallopian tube, causing a maternal hemorrhage.

Data Collection

- Risk Factors
  - Any factor that compromises tubal patency (pelvic inflammatory disease, contraceptive intrauterine device [IUD])

- Subjective Data
  - One or two missed menses
  - Unilateral stabbing pain and tenderness in the lower-abdominal quadrant
  - Scant, dark red, or brown vaginal spotting if tube ruptures (bleeding may be into the intraperitoneal area)
  - Referred shoulder pain from blood irritation of the diaphragm or phrenic nerve (common symptom)
  - Frequent nausea and vomiting after tube rupture

- Objective Data
  - Signs of hemorrhage and shock (hypotension, tachycardia, pallor)
  - Laboratory tests
    - Hormone levels of progesterone and hCG elevated
    - WBC count elevated to 15,000/mm3
  - Diagnostic procedures
    - Transvaginal ultrasound showing an empty uterus

Collaborative Care

- Nursing Care
  - Monitor clients receiving IV replacement fluids.
  - Monitor serum electrolytes.
  - Provide client education and psychological support.
  - Prepare clients for surgery and postoperative nursing care.

- Medication

  o Methotrexate (Rheumatrex)

  o Used to inhibit cell division and enlargement of the embryo. It also prevents rupture of the fallopian tube to preserve it.

  o Nursing considerations

    ▪ Obtain serum hCG levels, liver and renal function studies, CBC, blood type, and Rh-antibody status.

    ▪ Administer as single IM dose.

- Care After Discharge

  o Client education

    ▪ Instruct clients to avoid alcohol and vitamins containing folic acid to prevent a toxic response to the medication.

    ▪ Advise clients to minimize sun exposure (photosensitivity) by wearing sunscreen, long-sleeve shirts and pants, and a hat while outdoors.

    ▪ Instruct clients to return for a follow-up visit in one week for evaluation of hCG levels. Clients may need a second dose. Clients will need to have weekly evaluation of hCG levels until at expected level.

- Surgical interventions

  o Linear salpingostomy is done to salvage the fallopian tube if not ruptured.

  o Laparoscopic salpingostomy (removal of the tube) is performed when the tube has ruptured.

  o Client education

    ▪ Instruct clients to notify provider if pregnancy occurs to rule out recurrent ectopic pregnancy.

- Client Outcomes

  o The client will experience no physiological complications.

  o The client will have adequate psychological support to deal with the loss effectively.

GESTATIONAL TROPHOBLASTIC DISEASE (HYDATIDIFORM MOLE, CHORIOCARCINOMA, AND MOLAR PREGNANCY)

Overview

- Gestational trophoblastic disease is the proliferation and degeneration of trophoblastic villi in the placenta that becomes swollen, fluid-filled, and takes on the appearance of grape-like clusters. The embryo fails to develop beyond a primitive state and these structures are associated with choriocarcinoma, which is a rapidly metastasizing malignancy. Two types of molar growths are identified by chromosomal analysis.

- In the complete mole, all genetic material is paternally derived.

  o The ovum has no genetic material or the material is inactive.

  o The complete mole contains no fetus, placenta, amniotic membranes, or fluid.

  o There is no placenta to receive maternal blood; therefore, hemorrhage into the uterine cavity occurs and vaginal bleeding results.

  o Approximately 20% of complete moles progress toward a choriocarcinoma.

- In the partial mole, genetic material is derived both maternally and paternally.

  o A normal ovum is fertilized by two sperm or one sperm in which meiosis or chromosome reduction and division did not occur.

  o A partial mole often contains abnormal embryonic or fetal parts, an amniotic sac, and fetal blood, but congenital anomalies are present.

  o Approximately 6% of partial moles progress toward a choriocarcinoma.

Data Collection

- Risk Factors

  o Low protein intake

  o Under 18 years of age or older than 35 years of age

- Subjective Data

  o Vaginal bleeding at approximately 16 weeks of gestation

  o Excessive vomiting (hyperemesis gravidarum) due to elevated hCG levels

- Objective Data

  o Physical assessment findings

    ■ Rapid uterine growth larger than expected for the duration of the pregnancy due to the over proliferation of trophoblastic cells

    ■ Dark brown vaginal bleeding resembling prune juice, or bright red bleeding that is either scant or profuse and continues for a few days or intermittently for a few weeks

    ■ Bleeding accompanied by discharge from the clear fluid-filled vesicles

    ■ Findings are similar to gestational hypertension, including elevated blood pressure, edema, and proteinuria, which occur prior to 24 weeks of gestation

  o Laboratory tests

    ■ Urinalysis for proteinuria

      □ Serial hCG immunoassays for pregnancy are strongly positive (1 to 2 million IU compared with a normal pregnancy level of 400,000 IU), and secondary hCG is produced by the overgrowing trophoblastic cells.

- Analysis of serum hCG is performed every 1 to 2 weeks until levels are normal, every 2 to 4 weeks for 6 months, and every 2 months for 1 year. These analyses should be performed in this manner because levels that plateau or increase suggest a malignant transformation.
    - ○ Diagnostic procedures
        - An ultrasound will reveal a dense growth with characteristic vesicles, but no fetus in utero.

Collaborative Care

- Nursing Care

    - ○ Measure fundal height.

    - ○ Check for vaginal bleeding and discharge.

    - ○ Monitor gastrointestinal status and appetite.

    - ○ Check the client's extremities and face for edema.

- Medications

    - ○ Administer Rho(D) immune globulin (RhoGAM) to clients who are Rh-negative.

- Therapeutic Procedures

    - ○ Suction curettage is done to aspirate and evacuate the mole.

    - ○ Following mole evacuation, clients should undergo a baseline pelvic exam and ultrasound scan of the abdomen in addition to frequent follow-up pelvic exams.

- Care After Discharge

    - ○ Client education

        - Advise clients to bring any clots or tissue passed to the provider for evaluation.

        - Provide client education about the disease and emotional support regarding the loss of an anticipated pregnancy.

        - Instruct clients to use reliable contraception for 12 months because a pregnancy would make it impossible to monitor the decline in hCG levels, which is a significant component of follow-up care.

        - Instruct clients about the critical importance of follow-up because of the increased risk of choriocarcinoma.

- Client Outcomes

    - ○ The client will experience no physiological complications.

    - ○ The client will have adequate psychological support to deal with the loss effectively.

PLACENTA PREVIA

Overview

- Placenta previa occurs when the placenta abnormally implants in the lower segment of the uterus near or over the cervical os instead of attaching to the uterine fundus. The abnormal implantation results in bleeding during the third trimester of pregnancy as the cervix begins to dilate and efface.

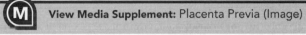

View Media Supplement: Placenta Previa (Image)

  - Placenta previa is classified into three types dependent on the degree to which the cervical os is covered by the placenta.
    - Complete or total – When the cervical os is completely covered by the placental attachment
    - Incomplete or partial – When the cervical os is only partially covered by the placental attachment
    - Marginal or low-lying – When the placenta is attached in the lower uterine segment but does not reach the cervical os

Data Collection

- Risk Factors
  - Previous placenta previa
  - Uterine scarring (previous cesarean birth, curettage, endometritis)
  - Maternal age greater than 35 years
  - Multifetal gestation
  - Multiple gestations or closely spaced pregnancies
- Subjective Data
  - Painless, bright red vaginal bleeding that increases as the cervix dilates
- Objective Data
  - Physical assessment findings
    - A soft, relaxed, nontender uterus with normal tone
    - A fundal height that is greater than usually expected for gestational age
    - A fetus in a breech, oblique, or transverse position
    - A palpable placenta
    - Vital signs within expected reference range
    - A decreasing urinary output

- o   Laboratory tests
    - ▪   Hgb and Hct for blood loss assessment
    - ▪   CBC
    - ▪   ABO blood typing and Rh-factor
    - ▪   Coagulation profile
    - ▪   Kleihauer-Betke test (used to detect fetal blood in maternal circulation)
- o   Diagnostic procedures
    - ▪   Transabdominal or transvaginal ultrasound for placement of the placenta
    - ▪   Fetal monitoring for fetal well-being assessment

Collaborative Care

- •   Nursing Care

    - o   Monitor clients for vaginal bleeding, leakage of amniotic fluid, or contractions.

    - o   Measure fundal height.

    - o   Perform Leopold's maneuvers to determine fetal position and presentation.

    - o   Refrain from performing vaginal exams (may exacerbate bleeding).

    - o   Monitor clients receiving IV fluids and blood transfusions.

    - o   Have oxygen equipment available in case of fetal distress.

- •   Medications

    - o   Corticosteroids such as betamethasone (Celestone) are prescribed for fetal lung maturation if delivery of the fetus is anticipated (cesarean birth).

- •   Therapeutic Procedures

    - o   Delivery of fetus by cesarean birth if previa is present at term gestation

- •   Care After Discharge

    - o   Client education
        - ▪   Instruct clients to follow activity restrictions such as bed rest.
        - ▪   Instruct clients to refrain from vaginal intercourse and not to insert anything vaginally.

- •   Client Outcomes

    - o   The client's pregnancy will be maintained without any maternal or fetal compromise.

ABRUPTIO PLACENTAE

 Overview

- Abruptio placentae is the premature separation of the placenta from the uterus, which can be a partial or complete detachment. This separation occurs after 20 weeks of gestation, which is usually in the third trimester. It has significant maternal and fetal morbidity and mortality and is a leading cause of maternal death.

> **(M)** **View Media Supplement:** Abruptio Placentae (Image)

  - Coagulation defect, such as disseminated intravascular coagulopathy (DIC), is often associated with moderate to severe abruption.

Data Collection

- Risk Factors

  - Maternal hypertension
  - Blunt external abdominal trauma (motor-vehicle crash, maternal battering)
  - Cocaine abuse resulting in vasoconstriction
  - Previous incidents of abruptio placentae
  - Cigarette smoking
  - Premature rupture of membranes
  - Multiple pregnancy

- Subjective Data

  - Sudden onset of intense localized uterine pain with vaginal bleeding

- Objective Data

  - Physical assessment findings
    - Vaginal bleeding that is bright red or dark
    - A board-like, tender abdomen
    - A firm, rigid uterus with contractions (uterine hypertonicity)
    - Fetal distress
    - Signs of hypovolemic shock
  - Laboratory tests
    - Hgb and Hct decreased
    - Coagulation factors decreased
    - Clotting defects DIC

- Cross and type match for possible blood transfusions
- Kleihauer-Betke test (used to detect fetal blood in maternal circulation)
  - Diagnostic procedures
    - Ultrasound for fetal well-being and placental assessment
    - Biophysical profile to ascertain fetal well-being

Collaborative Care

- Nursing Care
  - Palpate the uterus for tenderness and tone.
  - Monitor FHR pattern.
  - Refrain from vaginal exams (may exacerbate bleeding).
  - Monitor clients receiving IV fluids and blood transfusions.
  - Administer oxygen 8 to 10 L via face mask.
- Medications
  - Administer corticosteroids to promote fetal lung maturity.
- Therapeutic Procedures
  - Delivery of fetus if pregnancy is at term gestation; vaginally or by cesarean birth depending on degree of abruption
- Client Outcomes
  - The client and fetus will be free from injury.

VASA PREVIA

Overview

- A vasa previa is the presence of fetal blood vessels crossing the amniotic membranes over the cervical os. There is a high newborn mortality rate associated with this condition. The risk is associated with fetal hemorrhage, as the client's cervix dilates or membranes rupture.

- Diagnosing this condition during the antepartum period is associated with improved outcomes. However, this condition is rarely diagnosed prior to the onset of labor.

Data Collection

- Objective Data
  - Physical assessment findings
    - Painless heavy bleeding upon rupture of membranes
    - Fetal bradycardia

- ○ Laboratory tests
  - ▪ Hgb and Hct decreased
  - ▪ Cross and type match for possible blood transfusions
- ○ Diagnostic procedures
  - ▪ Confirmation by sonography

Collaborative Care

- • Nursing Care
  - ○ Monitor bleeding rate, amount, and color.
  - ○ Monitor clients receiving IV fluids and blood transfusions.
  - ○ Administer oxygen 8 to 10 L via face mask.
  - ○ Prepare for an emergency cesarean birth.
- • Care After Discharge
  - ○ Client education
    - ▪ Provide emotional support for clients and their families.
- • Client Outcomes
  - ○ The client and fetus will be free from injury.

Ⓐ APPLICATION EXERCISES

1. A nurse is reinforcing teaching to a client who has had a dilation and curettage to assist with termination of pregnancy following an incomplete abortion. Which of the following responses by the client indicates a need for further teaching

   A. "I will contact my doctor if I experience heavy, bright red vaginal bleeding."

   B. "I expect to have a small amount of discharge for 1 to 2 weeks."

   C. "I should refrain from sexual intercourse for 2 weeks."

   D. "I can get pregnant within 1 month."

2. A nurse at an antepartum clinic is caring for a client at 16 weeks of gestation diagnosed with a hydatidiform mole. Which of the following is an expected finding? (Select all that apply.)

   _____ Excessive vomiting

   _____ Scant prune-colored vaginal discharge

   _____ Increased fundal height measurement

   _____ Gestational hypertension

   _____ Polyuria

3. A nurse is providing care for a client diagnosed with a marginal abruptio placentae. The nurse is aware that which of the following findings are risk factors for developing this problem? (Select all that apply.)

   _____ Maternal hypertension

   _____ Blunt abdominal trauma

   _____ Cocaine abuse

   _____ Maternal age

   _____ Cigarette smoking

4. A nurse is providing care for a client who is diagnosed with an ectopic pregnancy. Which of the following medications should the nurse anticipate that the provider will prescribe?

   A. Betamethasone (Celestone)

   B. Indomethacin (Indocin)

   C. Methotrexate (Rheumatrex)

   D. Methylergonovine (Methergine)

5. A client presents to the birthing unit with painless bright red vaginal bleeding. The nurse is aware that these findings are associated with which of the following?

   A. Ectopic pregnancy

   B. Placenta previa

   C. Abruptio placentae

   D. Threatened abortion

Ⓐ APPLICATION EXERCISES ANSWER KEY

1. A nurse is reinforcing teaching to a client who has had a dilation and curettage to assist with termination of pregnancy following an incomplete abortion. Which of the following responses by the client indicates a need for further teaching

   A. "I will contact my doctor if I experience heavy, bright red vaginal bleeding."

   B. "I expect to have a small amount of discharge for 1 to 2 weeks."

   C. "I should refrain from sexual intercourse for 2 weeks."

   D. "I can get pregnant within 1 month."

   Pregnancy should be avoided for 2 months and the client will require additional teaching. The provider should be notified of heavy, bright red bleeding. A small amount of vaginal discharge is normal for 1 to 2 weeks. Refraining from sexual intercourse for 2 weeks is indicated.

   Ⓝ NCLEX® Connection: Reduction of Risk Potential, Potential for Alterations in Body Systems

2. A nurse at an antepartum clinic is caring for a client at 16 weeks of gestation diagnosed with a hydatidiform mole. Which of the following is an expected finding? (Select all that apply.)

X	**Excessive vomiting**
X	**Scant prune-colored vaginal discharge**
X	**Increased fundal height measurement**
X	**Gestational hypertension**
_____	Polyuria

   Hydatidiform mole (gestational trophoblastic disease) exhibits a uterine size that increases abnormally fast. The trophoblastic tissue causes abnormally high levels of hCG that result in excessive nausea and emesis. There is no fetus present on the ultrasound. There may be scant or profuse dark brown or red vaginal bleeding that first occurs in the second trimester, usually around 16 week of gestation. Hyperemesis gravidarum is accompanied by weight loss and dehydration. The client also exhibits symptoms of gestational hypertension including elevated blood pressure, edema, and proteinuria that occur prior to 20 weeks of gestation. Polyuria is not an expected finding with the diagnosis of hydatidiform mole.

   Ⓝ NCLEX® Connection: Physiological Adaptation, Alterations in Body Systems

3. A nurse is providing care for a client diagnosed with a marginal abruptio placentae. The nurse is aware that which of the following findings are risk factors for developing this problem? (Select all that apply.)

    __X__   **Maternal hypertension**

    __X__   **Blunt abdominal trauma**

    __X__   **Cocaine abuse**

    _____   Maternal age

    __X__   **Cigarette smoking**

Maternal hypertension, blunt abdominal trauma, cocaine abuse, and cigarette smoking are risk factors for abruptio placentae. Maternal age is not an associated risk for this condition. However, it is a risk factor for placenta previa.

 NCLEX® Connection: Physiological Adaptation, Alterations in Body Systems

4. A nurse is providing care for a client who is diagnosed with an ectopic pregnancy. Which of the following medications should the nurse anticipate that the provider will prescribe?

A. Betamethasone (Celestone)

B. Indomethacin (Indocin)

C. Methotrexate (Rheumatrex)

D. Methylergonovine (Methergine)

Methotrexate is prescribed to inhibit cell division and enlargement of the embryo in an ectopic pregnancy, and it also prevents rupture of the fallopian tube to preserve it. Corticosteroids are prescribed for fetal lung maturation if delivery of the fetus is anticipated. Indocin is used to treat preterm labor. Methergine is used to treat postpartum hemorrhage.

NCLEX® Connection: Pharmacological Therapies, Expected Actions/Outcomes

5. A client presents to the birthing unit with painless bright red vaginal bleeding. The nurse is aware that these findings are associated with which of the following?

A. Ectopic pregnancy

B. Placenta previa

C. Abruptio placentae

D. Threatened abortion

Painless vaginal bleeding is associated with placenta previa. An ectopic pregnancy is characterized by one or two missed menses, unilateral stabbing pain, and tenderness in the lower-abdominal quadrant, along with scant, dark red or brown vaginal spotting if a tube ruptures. Abruptio placentae is a condition with abdominal pain and either dark or bright red vaginal bleeding. A threatened abortion may have slight abdominal cramping with spotting to moderate vaginal bleeding.

NCLEX® Connection: Physiological Adaptation, Alterations in Body Systems

UNIT 1	ANTEPARTUM NURSING CARE
Section:	Complications of Pregnancy
Chapter 6	Infections

Overview

- Maternal infections during pregnancy require prompt identification and treatment. Infections that may affect pregnant clients include HIV, TORCH infections, streptococcus ß-hemolytic, Group B, chlamydia, gonorrhea, and *Candida albicans*.

HIV/AIDS

Overview

- HIV is a retrovirus that attacks and causes destruction of T lymphocytes. It causes immunosuppression in clients. HIV is transmitted from mothers to the fetus perinatally through the placenta and postnatally to newborns through the breast milk.

- Routine laboratory testing in the early prenatal period includes testing for HIV. Early identification and treatment significantly decreases the incidence of perinatal transmission.

- Testing is also recommended in the third trimester for clients who are at an increased risk.

- Use of internal fetal monitors, vacuum extraction, and forceps during labor should be avoided in clients who are HIV positive because of the risk of fetal bleeding.

- Injections and blood testing should not take place until the first bath is given to newborns of mothers who are HIV positive.

Data Collection

- Risk Factors

  - IV drug use

  - Multiple sexual partners

  - Bisexuality

  - Maternal history of multiple STIs

  - Blood transfusion (rare occurrence)

- Subjective Data

  o Fatigue

- Objective Data

  o Physical assessment findings

    ■ Diarrhea

    ■ Weight loss

    ■ Anemia

  o Laboratory tests

    ■ Testing begins with an antibody screening test such as enzyme immunoassay. Confirmation of positive results is confirmed by Western blot testing.

    ■ Screen clients for STIs such as gonorrhea, Chlamydia, syphilis, and hepatitis B.

    ■ Obtain frequent viral load levels and CD4 cell counts throughout the pregnancy of mothers who are HIV positive.

Collaborative Care

- Nursing Care

  o Provide support prior to and after testing.

  o Use standard precautions.

  o Administer antiviral combination therapy as prescribed.

- Medications

  o Retrovir (Zidovudine)

    ■ Antiretroviral agent

    ■ Nucleoside reverse transcriptase inhibitor

    ■ Nursing Considerations

      □ Start administration of retrovir after the first trimester and continue throughout the pregnancy.

      □ Administer retrovir to newborns following delivery and for 6 weeks following.

- Interdisciplinary care

  o Request referral for clients to a mental health counselor, legal assistance, and financial resources if indicated.

- Care After Discharge

  o Client education

    ▪ Instruct clients not to breastfeed.

    ▪ Discuss safe sexual relations with clients.

- Client Outcomes

  o The client will remain free from injury during pregnancy.

TORCH INFECTIONS

Overview

- TORCH is an acronym for a group of infections that can negatively affect women who are pregnant. These infections can cross the placenta and have teratogenic affects on the fetus.

Data Collection

- Risk Factors

  o Toxoplasmosis is caused by consumption of raw or undercooked meat or handling cat feces.

  o Rubella (German measles) is transmitted by droplet transmission of nasopharyngeal secretions of individuals who are infected. The virus is also present in blood, stool, and urine.

  o Cytomegalovirus (member of herpes virus family) is transmitted by droplet transmission and is found in semen, cervical and vaginal secretions, breast milk, placental tissue, urine, feces, and blood. Latent virus may be reactivated and cause disease to the fetus in utero or during passage through the birth canal.

  o Herpes simplex virus (HSV) is spread by direct contact with oral or genital lesions. Transmission to the fetus is greatest during vaginal birth if the woman has active lesions.

- Subjective Data

  o Toxoplasmosis symptoms similar to influenza or lymphadenopathy

    ▪ Reports of malaise, muscle aches, (flu-like symptoms)

  o Rubella

    ▪ Reports of joint and muscle pain

  o Cytomegalovirus is usually asymptomatic.

  o Herpes simplex virus

    ▪ Reports of dysuria, malaise, fever, chills and numerous painful genital lesions

- Objective Data

  - Physical assessment findings

    - Signs of toxoplasmosis include fever and tender lymph nodes.

    - Signs of rubella include rash, mild lymphedema, fever, and fetal consequences, which include miscarriage, congenital anomalies, and death.

    - Herpes simplex virus initially presents with macules and papules that progress to purulent vesicles.

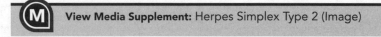

View Media Supplement: Herpes Simplex Type 2 (Image)

  - Laboratory tests

    - For herpes simplex, obtain cultures from women who have HSV or are at or near term.

  - Diagnostic procedures

    - A TORCH screen is an immunologic survey that is used to identify the existence of these infections in mothers (to identify fetal risks) or in newborns (detection of antibodies against infections).

Collaborative Care

- Nursing Care

  - Monitor fetal well-being.

  - Educate clients on prevention practices including good hand hygiene and cooking meat properly.

- Medications

  - Administer antibiotics as prescribed.

  - For toxoplasmosis treatment, include sulfonamides or a combination of pyrimethamine and sulfadiazine (potentially harmful to the fetus, but parasitic treatment essential).

- Care After Discharge

  - Client education

    - Instruct pregnant clients with rubella to avoid groups of young children.

    - Encourage clients with low rubella titers to receive immunizations prior to their next pregnancy (usually done prior to discharge from the hospital after delivery). Clients need to wait 4 weeks after immunization to become pregnant.

    - Reinforce the need for clients to adhere to the complete prescribed treatment.

    - Provide clients with emotional support.

- Client Outcomes

  o Clients will be free of clinical findings indicating viral complications are affecting the pregnancy.

STREPTOCOCCUS BETA-HEMOLYTIC, GROUP B

 Overview

- Streptococcus ß-hemolytic, Group B (GBS) is a bacterial infection that can be passed to newborns during labor and delivery.

Data Collection

- Risk Factors

  o History of positive culture with previous pregnancy

  o Risk factors for neonatal GBS

    - Positive culture with pregnancy

    - Prolonged rupture of membranes

    - Preterm delivery

- Objective Data

  o Physical assessment findings

    - Positive GBS may have maternal and fetal effects including premature rupture of membranes, preterm labor and delivery, chorioamnionitis, infections of the urinary tract, and maternal sepsis.

  o Laboratory tests

    - Vaginal and rectal cultures are performed between 35 to 37 weeks of gestation.

Collaborative Care

- Nursing Care

  o Administer prophylaxis antibiotics during labor.

- Medications

  o Penicillin G or ampicillin (Principen) may be prescribed as intermittent IV bolus to treat positive GBS.

- Care After Discharge

  o Client education

    - Instruct clients to monitor for signs of infection and to report to the provider.

- Client Outcomes

  o The newborn's blood culture is negative for GBS with no clinical signs of sepsis.

CHLAMYDIA

Overview

- Chlamydia is a bacterial infection caused by Chlamydia trachomatis. It is the most common STI. The infection is often difficult to diagnose because it is typically asymptomatic. According to current guidelines from the Centers for Disease Control and Prevention, all women and adolescents ages 20 to 25 who are sexually active should be screened for STIs.

Data Collection

- Risk Factors

  o Multiple sexual partners

  o Unprotected sexual practices

- Subjective Data

  o Vaginal spotting

  o Vulvar itching

- Objective Data

  o Physical assessment findings

    ▪ White, watery vaginal discharge

  o Laboratory tests

    ▪ Endocervical culture

Collaborative Care

- Nursing Care

  o Instruct clients to take the entire prescription as prescribed.

  o Identify and treat all sexual partners.

  o Retest clients who are pregnant in 3 weeks after completing the prescribed regimen.

- Medications

  o Azithromycin (Zithromax), amoxicillin (Amoxil), and erythromycin (Ery-Tab) are prescribed during pregnancy.

    ▪ Broad-spectrum antibiotic

    ▪ Bactericidal action

- Nursing Considerations
  - □ Administer 0.5% erythromycin ophthalmic ointment to all newborns following delivery. This antibiotic is both bacteriostatic and bactericidal, thus it provides prophylaxis against Neisseria gonorrhoeae and Chlamydia trachomatis.

- Care After Discharge

  - Client education

    - Instruct clients to take all prescription as prescribed.

    - Educate clients about the possibility of decreasing effectiveness of oral contraceptives.

- Client Outcomes

  - The client will be free of clinical findings of infection.

GONORRHEA

 Overview

- Neisseria gonorrhoeae is the causative agent of gonorrhea. Gonorrhea is a bacterial infection that is primarily spread by genital-to-genital contact. However, it can also be spread by anal-to-genital contact or oral-to-genital contact. It can also be transmitted to a neonate during delivery. Women are frequently asymptomatic.

Data Collection

- Risk Factors

  - Multiple sexual partners

  - Unprotected sexual practices

- Subjective Data (Male)

  - Urethral discharge

  - Painful urination

  - Frequency

- Subjective Data (Female)

  - Lower abdominal pain

  - Dysmenorrhea

- Objective Data – Male/Female

  - Physical assessment findings

    - Urethral discharge

    - Yellowish-green vaginal discharge

- Reddened vulva and vaginal walls
- If gonorrhea is left untreated, it can cause pelvic inflammatory disease, heart disease, and arthritis.
    - Laboratory tests
        - Urethral and vaginal cultures
        - Urine culture

Collaborative Care

- Nursing Care
    - Provide clients education regarding disease transmission.
    - Instruct clients to take the entire prescription as prescribed.
    - Identify and treat all sexual partners.
- Medications
    - Ceftriaxone (Rocephin) IM or azithromycin (Zithromax) PO
        - Given for 7 days
        - Broad-spectrum antibiotic
        - Bactericidal action
- Care After Discharge
    - Client education
        - Instruct clients to finish all prescribed medications.
        - Instruct clients to repeat the culture to assess for medication effectiveness.
        - Educate clients regarding safe-sex practices.
- Client Outcomes
    - The client will be free of clinical findings of infection.

CANDIDA ALBICANS

Overview

- A fungal infection caused by *Candida albicans*.

Data Collection

- Risk Factors
    - Diabetes mellitus
    - Oral contraceptives
    - Recent antibiotic treatment

- Subjective Data

  o Vulvar itching

- Objective Data

  o Physical assessment findings

    ■ Thick, creamy white vaginal discharge

    ■ Vulvar redness

    ■ White patches on vaginal walls

    ■ Gray-white patches on the tongue and gums (newborns)

  o Laboratory tests

    ■ Wet prep

  o Diagnostic procedures

    ■ Potassium hydroxide (KOH) prep

    ■ Presence of hyphae and pseudohyphae indicates positive findings

Collaborative Care

- Nursing Care

  o Medications

    ■ Over-the-counter treatments, such as clotrimazole (Gyne-Lotrimin) or miconazole (Monistat), are available to treat candidiasis. However, it is important for the provider to diagnosis candidiasis initially.

- Care After Discharge

  o Client education

    ■ Administer medication as prescribed.

- Client Outcomes

  o The client will be free of clinical findings of infection.

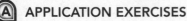

APPLICATION EXERCISES

1. A nurse is admitting a client in labor to the obstetrical unit. The client has a positive human immunodeficiency virus (HIV) status. Discuss the contraindications for this client.

2. A nurse in an antepartum clinic is providing care for a client. Which of the following clinical findings are suggestive of gonorrhea? (Select all that apply.)

   _____ Dysmenorrhea

   _____ Yellowish-green vaginal discharge

   _____ Reddened vulva

   _____ Malaise

   _____ Lower abdominal pain

3. A nurse is caring for a pregnant client diagnosed with chlamydia. Which of the following medications does the nurse anticipate the provider will prescribe? (Select all that apply.)

   _____ Ceftriaxone (Rocephin)

   _____ Azithromycin (Zithromax)

   _____ Amoxicillin (Amoxil)

   _____ Metronidazole (Flagyl)

   _____ Erythromycin (Ery-Tab)

4. A nurse is caring for a pregnant client diagnosed with human immunodeficiency virus (HIV). Which of the following medications does the nurse anticipate the provider will prescribe?

   A. Ceftriaxone (Rocephin)

   B. Retrovir (Zidovudine)

   C. Metronidazole (Flagyl)

   D. Tetracycline (Sumycin)

5. A nurse in an antepartum clinic is reviewing the laboratory reports of several clients. The nurse is aware that which of the following infections have medications that can be prescribed as prophylactic treatment during labor or immediately following delivery? (Select all that apply.)

   _____ Gonorrhea

   _____ Chlamydia

   _____ HIV

   _____ Group B Strep

   _____ TORCH

APPLICATION EXERCISES ANSWER KEY

1. A nurse is admitting a client in labor to the obstetrical unit. The client has a positive human immunodeficiency virus (HIV) status. Discuss the contraindications for this client.

   Episiotomy is contraindicated for HIV-positive clients due to the risk of maternal blood exposure. Additionally, the use of internal fetal monitors, vacuum extraction, and forceps during labor should be avoided because of the risk of fetal bleeding.

    NCLEX® Connection: Physiological Adaptation, Alterations in Body Systems

2. A nurse in an antepartum clinic is providing care for a client. Which of the following clinical findings are suggestive of gonorrhea? (Select all that apply.)

X	**Dysmenorrhea**
X	**Yellowish-green vaginal discharge**
X	**Reddened vulva**
	Malaise
X	**Lower abdominal pain**

   Symptoms of gonorrhea include reports of dysmenorrhea and lower abdominal pain. Objective findings include yellowish-green vaginal discharge and reddened vulva and vaginal walls. Malaise is not a clinical finding associated with gonorrhea.

    NCLEX® Connection: Physiological Adaptation, Alterations in Body Systems

3. A nurse is caring for a pregnant client diagnosed with chlamydia. Which of the following medications does the nurse anticipate the provider will prescribe? (Select all that apply.)

	Ceftriaxone (Rocephin)
X	**Azithromycin (Zithromax)**
X	**Amoxicillin (Amoxil)**
	Metronidazole (Flagyl)
X	**Erythromycin (Ery-Tab)**

   Azithromycin, amoxicillin, and erythromycin are prescribed during pregnancy to treat Chlamydia.

    NCLEX® Connection: Pharmacological Therapies, Expected Actions/Outcomes

4. A nurse is caring for a pregnant client diagnosed with human immunodeficiency virus (HIV). Which of the following medications does the nurse anticipate the provider will prescribe?

    A. Ceftriaxone (Rocephin)

    B. Retrovir (Zidovudine)

    C. Metronidazole (Flagyl)

    D. Tetracycline (Sumycin)

Retrovir (Zidovudine) is prescribed for the treatment of HIV. Start administration of retrovir after the first trimester and continue throughout the pregnancy. Additionally, it is prescribed to the neonate following delivery and for 6 weeks. Ceftriaxone (Rocephin) IM is prescribed for the treatment of gonorrhea. Metronidazole (Flagyl) is used in the treatment of bacterial vaginosis and trichomoniasis. Tetracycline (Sumycin) is used to treat syphilis.

Ⓝ NCLEX® Connection: Physiological Adaptation, Alterations in Body Systems

5. A nurse in an antepartum clinic is reviewing the laboratory reports of several clients. The nurse is aware that which of the following infections have medications that can be prescribed as prophylactic treatment during labor or immediately following delivery? (Select all that apply.)

    __X__   **Gonorrhea**

    __X__   **Chlamydia**

    __X__   **HIV**

    __X__   **Group B Strep**

    _____   TORCH

Erythromycin is the medication of choice for ophthalmia neonatorum. This antibiotic is both bacteriostatic and bactericidal, thus providing prophylaxis against Neisseria gonorrhoeae and Chlamydia trachomatis. It is administrated to the neonate immediately following delivery. Retrovir (Zidovudine) is prescribed to the client in labor who is HIV positive. It is also administered to the newborn following delivery and for 6 weeks thereafter. Penicillin G or ampicillin may be prescribed to treat positive GBS.

Ⓝ NCLEX® Connection: Physiological Adaptation, Alterations in Body Systems

UNIT 1	ANTEPARTUM NURSING CARE
Section:	Complications of Pregnancy
Chapter 7	Clinical Disorders

Overview

- Unexpected medical conditions may occur during pregnancy. Awareness, early detection, and interventions are crucial components to ensure fetal well-being and maternal health.

- Unexpected medical conditions include incompetent cervix, hyperemesis gravidarum, anemia, gestational diabetes mellitus, gestational hypertension, preeclampsia, and heart disease.

INCOMPETENT CERVIX

Overview

- Incompetent cervix is the painless dilation of the cervix in the absence of uterine contractions. The cervix is incapable of supporting the weight and pressure of the growing fetus and results in expulsion of the products of conception during the second trimester of pregnancy. This usually occurs around 20 weeks of gestation.

Data Collection

- Risk Factors

    o History of cervical trauma (previous lacerations, excessive dilations or cervical biopsy)

    o In utero, exposure to diethylstilbestrol (DES) (ingested by the client's mother during pregnancy)

    o Congenital structural defects

    o Increased maternal age

- Subjective Data

    o Increase in pelvic pressure

- Objective Data

    o Physical assessment findings

        ▪ Pink-stained vaginal discharge or bleeding

        ▪ Possible gush of fluid (rupture of membranes)

- Uterine contractions with the expulsion of the fetus

- Postoperative (cerclage) monitoring for uterine contractions, rupture of membranes, and signs of infection

○ Diagnostic procedures

- An ultrasound showing a short cervix (less than 20 mm in length) indicates a reduced cervical competence.

- Prophylactic cervical cerclage is the surgical reinforcement of the cervix with a heavy ligature that is placed submucosally around the cervix to strengthen it and prevent premature cervical dilation. The cerclage is removed at 37 weeks of gestation.

Collaborative Care

- Nursing Care

  ○ Evaluate the client's support systems and availability of assistance if activity restrictions and/or bed rest are prescribed.

  ○ Check vaginal discharge.

  ○ Monitor the client's reports of pressure and contractions.

  ○ Monitor the client's vital signs

- Medications

  ○ Monitor clients receiving tocolytics prophylactically to inhibit uterine contractions.

- Care After Discharge

  ○ Client education

    - Instruct clients on activity restriction/bed rest as prescribed by the health care provider.

    - Encourage clients to maintain adequate hydration to promote a relaxed uterus (dehydration stimulates uterine contractions).

    - Advise clients to refrain from intercourse, prolonged standing for more than 90 min, and heavy lifting.

    - Instruct clients to report the rupture of membranes, strong-smelling vaginal discharge, mild uterine contractions less than 5 min apart, severe perineal pressure, and an urge to push.

    - Instruct clients on how to use the home uterine activity monitor in order to monitor for uterine contractions.

    - Arrange for clients to follow up with a home-health agency for observation and supervision.

    - Instruct clients that the cerclage should be removed around 37 weeks of gestation.

- Client Outcomes

  o The client will remain free of injury during pregnancy.

  o The client will maintain the pregnancy until term.

HYPEREMESIS GRAVIDARUM

Overview

- Hyperemesis gravidarum is excessive nausea and vomiting (related to elevated hCG levels) that is present beyond 12 weeks of gestation and results in a 5% weight loss from prepregnancy weight, electrolyte imbalance, ketonuria, and ketosis.

- Hyperemesis gravidarum may be present with liver dysfunction.

- There is a risk to the fetus for intrauterine growth restriction (IUGR) or preterm birth if the condition persists.

Data Collection

- Risk Factors

  o Maternal age younger than 20 years

  o Obesity

  o First pregnancy

  o Multifetal gestation

  o Gestational trophoblastic disease

  o Women with a history of psychiatric disorders

  o Transient hyperthyroidism

  o Vitamin B deficiencies

  o High stress levels

- Subjective Data

  o Reports of nausea and vomiting lasting past 12 weeks of gestation

  o Reports of excessive vomiting for prolonged periods

- Objective Data

  o Physical assessment findings

    ■ Weight loss

    ■ Increased pulse rate

    ■ Decreased blood pressure

    ■ Poor skin turgor

- ○ Laboratory tests
  - Urinalysis for ketones and acetones (breakdown of protein and fat)
  - Elevated specific gravity
  - Chemistry profile revealing electrolyte imbalances such as:
    - □ Decreased sodium, potassium, and chloride
    - □ Acidosis
    - □ Elevated liver enzymes
  - Thyroid test indicating hyperthyroidism
  - Increased Hct

Collaborative Care

- Nursing Care
  - ○ Monitor I&O.
  - ○ Check skin turgor and mucus membranes.
  - ○ Monitor vital signs and weight.
  - ○ Maintain NPO for 24 to 48 hr.
  - ○ Monitor IV fluids (isotonic solution such as lactated Ringer's).
  - ○ Administer enteral nutrition via NG tube if indicated.
  - ○ Monitor clients receiving total parental nutrition (TPN).
  - ○ Provide clear fluids after 24 hr if no vomiting.
  - ○ Advance the client's diet, as tolerated, with frequent, small meals. Start with dry toast, crackers, or cereal.
- Medications
  - ○ Give pyridoxine (Vitamin B_6) and other vitamin supplements as tolerated.
  - ○ Use antiemetic medications cautiously for uncontrollable nausea and vomiting (promethazine [Phenergan], metoclopramide [Reglan]).
  - ○ Use corticosteroids to treat refractory hyperemesis gravidarum.
- Care After Discharge
  - ○ Client education
    - Encourage clients to:
      - □ Get adequate rest.
      - □ Drink 2 to 3 L/day of fluids from food and beverage sources.
      - □ Eat small, frequent meals.

- Instruct clients to report return of clinical findings.
- Client Outcomes
  - The client will maintain
    - Fluid and electrolyte balance.
    - Adequate nutritional intake for pregnancy.
    - Adequate weight gain for pregnancy.

ANEMIA

 Overview

- Iron-deficiency anemia occurs during pregnancy due to inadequate maternal iron stores, consuming insufficient amounts of dietary iron, and hemodilution.

Data Collection

- Risk Factors
  - Less than 2 years between pregnancies
  - Heavy menses
  - Diet low in iron
- Subjective Data
  - Fatigue
  - Irritability
  - Headache
  - Shortness of breath with exertion
  - Palpitations
  - Craving to ingest any material not considered food (pica), such as starch, clay, soap, etc.
- Objective Data
  - Physical assessment findings
    - Pallor
    - Brittle nails
    - Shortness of breath
  - Laboratory tests
    - Hgb less than 12 mg/dL
    - Hct less than 33%

Collaborative Care

- Nursing Care

  - Instruct clients to increase dietary intake of foods rich in iron (legumes, fruit, green, leafy vegetables, and meat).

  - Educate clients about ways to minimize gastrointestinal side effects.

- Medications

  - Ferrous sulfate iron supplements

    - Used to increase Hgb and Hct levels

    - Nursing considerations and client education

      - Instruct the client to take the supplement on an empty stomach.

      - Instruct the client to take with vitamin C (orange juice) to increase absorption.

      - Suggest that clients increase fiber in their diet to assist with the discomforts of constipation.

  - Iron dextran (Imferon)

    - Used in the treatment of iron-deficiency anemia when oral iron supplements cannot be tolerated by clients who are pregnant

- Client Outcomes

  - The client will maintain Hgb and Hct levels within the expected reference range.

GESTATIONAL DIABETES MELLITUS

Overview

- Gestational diabetes mellitus presents as an impaired tolerance to glucose with the first onset or recognition during pregnancy. The ideal blood glucose level during pregnancy is 70 to 110 mg/dL.

- Gestational diabetes mellitus causes increased risks to the fetus including:

  - Spontaneous abortion, which is related to poor glycemic control.

  - Infections (urinary and vaginal), which are related to increased glucose in the urine and decreased resistance to infection because of altered carbohydrate metabolism.

  - Hydramnios, which can cause overdistention of the uterus, premature rupture of membranes, preterm labor, and hemorrhage.

  - Ketoacidosis from diabetogenic effect of pregnancy (increased insulin resistance), untreated hyperglycemia, or inappropriate insulin dosing.

  - Hypoglycemia, which is caused by overdosing in insulin, skipped or late meals, or increased exercise.

  - Hyperglycemia, which can cause excessive fetal growth (macrosomia).

Data Collection

- Risk Factors

  - Obesity

  - Maternal age older than 25 years

  - Family history of diabetes mellitus

  - Previous delivery of an infant that was large or stillborn

- Subjective Data

  - Reports of nervousness, headache, weakness, lightheadedness, irritability, hunger, blurred vision (hypoglycemia)

  - Reports of thirst, weakness, malaise, frequent urination (hyperglycemia)

- Objective Data

  - Physical assessment findings

    - Blood glucose less than expected reference range (hypoglycemia)

      - Hunger, lightheadedness, and shakiness

      - Nausea

      - Anxiety and irritability

      - Confusion

      - Slurred speech, decreased level of consciousness

      - Diaphoresis

      - Clammy pale skin

      - Respirations that are unchanged

      - Rapid pulse and palpitations

      - Headache and blurred vision

    - Blood glucose greater than expected reference range (hyperglycemia)

      - Thirst, frequent urination, hunger

      - Flushed, warm, dry skin

      - Rapid, deep respirations (Kussmaul respirations, with acetone/fruity odor due to ketones)

      - Rapid, weak pulse, hypotension

      - Excess weight gain during pregnancy

      - Weakness, malaise

- o Laboratory tests

  - ▪ Routine urinalysis with glycosuria

  - ▪ A Glucola screening test/1 hr glucose tolerance test (50 g oral glucose load, followed by plasma glucose analysis 1 hr later performed at 24 to 28 weeks of gestation – fasting not necessary; a positive blood glucose screening is 140 mg/dL or greater; additional testing with a 3-hr glucose tolerance test if indicated)

  - ▪ A 3-hr glucose tolerance test (following overnight fasting, avoidance of caffeine, and abstinence from smoking for 12 hr prior to testing; a fasting glucose is obtained, a 100 g glucose load is given, and serum glucose levels are determined at 1, 2, and 3 hr following glucose ingestion)

  - ▪ Ketones tested to assess the severity of ketoacidosis

- o Diagnostic procedures

  - ▪ Biophysical profile

  - ▪ Amniocentesis to include alpha-fetoprotein

  - ▪ Nonstress test

Collaborative Care

- Nursing Care

  - o Monitor the client's blood glucose.

  - o Instruct the client to perform daily kick counts.

- Medications

  - o Administer insulin as prescribed.

    - ▪ Most oral hypoglycemic agents are contraindicated for gestational diabetes mellitus, but there is limited use of glyburide (DiaBeta) at this time. The provider will need to make the determination if these medications may be used.

- Care After Discharge

  - o Client education

    - ▪ Educate clients about diet and exercise.

    - ▪ Instruct clients about glucose testing and self-administration of insulin.

    - ▪ Educate clients about signs of hypo- and hyperglycemia and appropriate treatment.

- Client Outcomes

  - o The client will effectively manage and control blood glucose level throughout her pregnancy to ensure maternal/fetal well-being.

GESTATIONAL HYPERTENSION/PREECLAMPSIA

Overview

- Hypertensive disease in pregnancy is divided into clinical subsets of the disease based on end-organ effects and can progress along a continuum from mild gestational hypertension to mild and/or severe preeclampsia, to eclampsia, to HELLP syndrome (hemolysis), elevated liver enzymes, and low platelets).

Gestational hypertension (GH),	<ul><li>Begins after the 20th week of pregnancy</li><li>Blood pressure of 140/90 mm Hg or greater, or a systolic increase of 30 mm Hg or a diastolic increase of 15 mm Hg from the prepregnancy baseline</li><li>No proteinuria or edema</li><li>Blood pressure returns to baseline by 12 weeks postpartum</li></ul>
Mild preeclampsia	<ul><li>Begins after the 20th week of pregnancy</li><li>Blood pressure of 140/90 mm Hg or greater, or a systolic increase of 30 mm Hg or a diastolic increase of 15 mm Hg from 1 to 2+ proteinuria</li><li>Weight gain of more than 2 kg (4.4 lb) per week in the second and third trimesters</li><li>Mild edema in upper extremities or face</li></ul>
Severe preeclampsia	<ul><li>Blood pressure of 160/100 mm Hg or greater</li><li>Proteinuria 3 to 4+</li><li>Oliguria</li><li>Elevated serum creatinine greater than 1.2 mg/dL</li><li>Cerebral or visual disturbances (headache and blurred vision)</li><li>Hyperreflexia with possible ankle clonus</li><li>Pulmonary, cardiac, or hepatic involvement</li><li>Extensive peripheral edema</li><li>Epigastric and right upper-quadrant pain</li><li>Thrombocytopenia</li></ul>
Eclampsia	<ul><li>Severe preeclampsia with onset of seizure activity or coma</li></ul>

- HELLP syndrome is a variant of severe preeclampsia in which hematologic conditions and hepatic dysfunction coexist. HELLP syndrome is diagnosed by laboratory tests, not clinically.

  o H – hemolysis resulting in anemia and jaundice

  o EL – elevated liver enzymes resulting in elevated alanine aminotransferase (ALT) or aspartate transaminase (AST), epigastric pain, and nausea and vomiting

  o LP – low platelets (< 100,000/mm³), resulting in thrombocytopenia, abnormal bleeding and clotting time, bleeding gums, petechiae, and possibly DIC

- Gestational hypertensive disease and chronic hypertension may occur simultaneously

- Gestational hypertensive diseases are associated with placental abruption, acute renal failure, hepatic rupture, preterm birth, and fetal and maternal death

Data Collection

- Risk Factors

  o No single profile identifies risks for gestational hypertensive disorders, but some high risks include:

    ▪ Maternal age younger than 20 or older than 40

    ▪ First pregnancy

    ▪ Morbid obesity

    ▪ Multifetal gestation

    ▪ Chronic renal disease

    ▪ Chronic hypertension

    ▪ Familiar history of preeclampsia

    ▪ Diabetes mellitus

    ▪ Rh incompatibility

    ▪ Molar pregnancy

    ▪ Previous history of GH

- Subjective Data

  o Severe continuous headache

  o Nausea

  o Blurring of vision

  o Flashes of lights or dots before the eyes

- Objective Data
  - ○ Physical assessment findings
    - Hypertension
    - Proteinuria
    - Periorbital, facial, hand, and abdominal edema
    - Pitting edema of lower extremities
    - Vomiting
    - Oliguria
    - Hyperreflexia
    - Scotoma
    - Epigastric pain
    - Right-upper quadrant pain
    - Dyspnea
    - Diminished breath sounds
    - Seizures
    - Jaundice
    - Rapid weight gain (2 kg [4.4 lb]) per week in the second and third trimesters
  - ○ Abnormal laboratory findings
    - Elevated liver enzymes (ALT, AST)
    - Increased serum creatinine
    - Increased plasma uric acid
    - Thrombocytopenia
    - Decreased Hgb
    - Hyperbilirubinemia
  - ○ Laboratory tests
    - Liver enzymes
    - Serum creatinine, BUN, uric acid, and magnesium increase as renal function decreases
    - CBC
    - Clotting studies
    - Chemistry profile
  - ○ Diagnostic procedures
    - Dipstick testing of urine for proteinuria
    - Twenty-four hour urine collection for protein and creatinine clearance

- Nonstress test, contraction stress test, biophysical profile, and serial ultrasounds to assess fetal status
- Doppler blood flow analysis to assess fetal well-being

Collaborative Care

- Nursing Care
  - Monitor level of consciousness.
  - Monitor vital signs including pulse oximetry.
  - Monitor the client's urine output and obtain a clean-catch urine sample to check for proteinuria.
  - Obtain daily weights.
  - Maintain clients on bed rest.
  - Promote divisional activities.
  - Encourage clients to maintain side-lying position.
  - Perform NST and daily kick counts as prescribed.
  - Maintain a dark quiet environment to avoid stimuli that may precipitate a seizure.
  - Limit visitors.
  - Maintain a patent airway in the event of a seizure.
  - Administer antihypertensive medications as prescribed.
- Medications
  - Magnesium sulfate
    - Anticonvulsant, antihypertensive, and CNS depressant
  - Nursing considerations

  - Monitor clients receiving magnesium sulfate by IV infusion.
  - Insert indwelling urinary catheter.
  - Monitor clients for signs of magnesium sulfate toxicity.
    - Absence of patellar deep tendon reflexes
    - Urine output less than 30 mL/hr
    - Respirations less than 12/min
    - Decreased level of consciousness
    - Cardiac dysrhythmias
  - Have calcium gluconate readily available for treatment of toxicity.
    - Monitor clients receiving calcium gluconate for magnesium toxicity.

- Care After Discharge

  o Client education

    ▪ Instruct clients to avoid foods that are high in sodium.

    ▪ Avoid alcohol and limit caffeine intake.

    ▪ Consume 2 to 3 L/day of fluids from food and beverage sources.

- Client Outcomes

  o The client will maintain blood pressure within acceptable parameters.

  o The client and fetus will remain free of injury.

HEART DISEASE

Overview

- Cardiovascular disease in pregnancy warrants early identification and monitoring to decrease incidence of maternal or fetal complications. Congenital cardiac anomaly and valvular disorders are the most common cardiovascular diseases seen in clients who are pregnant.

NEW YORK HEART ASSOCIATION'S CLASSIFICATION OF HEART DISEASE	
• Class I	• Client exhibits no symptoms with activity
• Class II	• Client has symptoms with ordinary exertion
• Class III	• Client displays symptoms with minimal exertion
• Class IV	• Client has symptoms at rest

- The above classification system will guide the provider in the management of cardiovascular disease during the antepartum, intrapartum, and postpartum periods and assist with predicting client outcomes.

- The provider will evaluate the client's classification at 3 and 7 months gestation to determine appropriate treatment and interventions.

- Clients meeting classification I and II should experience a normal pregnancy and delivery. Total bed rest is indicated for clients in classification III. Clients within classification IV are not good candidates for pregnancy and all risk factors should be discussed with the client.

Data Collection

- At risk for:

  o Preterm labor

  o Miscarriage

  o Intrauterine growth restriction

- Subjective Data
  - Dizziness
  - Shortness of breath
  - Weakness
  - Fatigue
  - Chest pain on exertion
  - Anxiety
- Objective Data
  - Physical assessment findings
    - Arrhythmias
    - Irregular heart rate
    - Tachycardia
    - Heart murmur
    - Distended jugular veins
    - Cyanosis of nails or lips
    - Pallor
    - Generalized edema
    - Diaphoresis
    - Increased respirations
    - Cough
    - Hemoptysis
    - Intrauterine growth restriction
    - Decreased amniotic fluid
    - FHR with decreased variability
  - Laboratory tests
    - CBC
    - Chemistry profile
    - Sedimentation rate
    - Maternal ABGs
    - Clotting studies
  - Diagnostic procedures
    - Echocardiogram
    - Holter monitoring

- Chest x-ray
- Ultrasound
- Pulse oximetry
- NST
- Biophysical profile

Collaborative Care

- Nursing Care

  o Instruct clients to adhere to bed rest.

  o Provide clients with education related to restricting dietary sodium intake and adhering to a cardiac diet.

  o Instruct clients to decrease physical activity.

  o Monitor vital signs.

  o Monitor FHR and uterine contractions.

  o Administer influenza and pneumococcus vaccines.

  o Encourage clients to take prenatal vitamins and iron supplements.

  o Administer oxygen to clients as prescribed.

  o Monitor the client's daily weight and urinary output.

  o Perform diagnostic procedures and laboratory studies as indicated.

  o Instruct the client to perform daily kick counts to assess fetal well-being.

  o Perform NST as prescribed.

- Medications – Pharmacological management is determined by the client's cardiac diagnoses and clinical presentation.

  o Propranolol (Inderal)

    - Beta blocker
    - Used to treat tachyarrhythmias and to lower maternal blood pressure

  o Gentamicin (Garamycin)

    - Aminoglycoside antibiotic
    - Prophylaxis that is given to prevent endocarditis

  o Ampicillin (Polycillin)

    - Antibiotic
    - Prophylaxis that is given to prevent endocarditis

- o Heparin sodium
  - Anticoagulant
  - Used in treating clients with pulmonary embolus, deep vein thrombosis, prosthetic valves, cyanotic heart defects, and rheumatic heart disease
- o Digoxin (Lanoxin)
  - Cardiac glycoside
  - Used to increase cardiac output during pregnancy, and may be prescribed if fetal tachycardia is present

- Interdisciplinary Care

  - o Request a referral for a dietician to assist with appropriate food choices.

  - o Consult with a cardiologist to monitor and treat cardiac status.

  - o Consult with a maternal/fetal specialist for collaborative management of high-risk pregnancy.

- Care After Discharge

  - o Client education

    - Instruct clients to notify the provider of clinical findings of infection.

    - Reinforce education related to medication therapy.

    - Instruct clients to perform daily kick counts.

- Client Outcomes

  - o The client will:

    - Remain free of injury during pregnancy.

    - Be free of infection.

    - Maintain adequate cardiac function to sustain pregnancy.

    - Be free of complications related to cardiac function.

- Complications

  - o Clients with cardiac disease may experience complications including right-sided heart failure, hypertension, arrhythmias, pulmonary hypertension, heart failure, aneurysm, aortic dissection, and maternal/fetal death.

Ⓐ APPLICATION EXERCISES

1. A nurse is caring for a client at 13 weeks of gestation who is diagnosed with hyperemesis gravidarum. The nurse is aware that which of the following is a risk factor for the client?

    A. Maternal age greater than 40

    B. Vitamin B deficiencies

    C. Oligohydramnios

    D. Placenta previa

2. A nurse in the antepartum clinic is collecting data for a client who is diagnosed with gestational diabetes mellitus. Which of the following findings indicate hyperglycemia? (Select all that apply.)

    _____ Flushed dry skin

    _____ Fruity breath odor

    _____ Hypotension

    _____ Slurred speech

    _____ Diaphoresis

3. A nurse is assisting with the care of a client diagnosed with preeclampsia and is prescribed an IV infusion of magnesium sulfate. The nurse is aware that which of the following medications should be available in the event of magnesium sulfate toxicity?

    A. Calcium gluconate

    B. Oxytocin (Pitocin)

    C. Terbutaline (Brethine)

    D. Misoprostol (Cytotec)

4. The nurse should monitor for which of the following signs of magnesium sulfate toxicity? (Select all that apply.)

    _____ Respirations less than 12/min

    _____ Urinary output less than 30 mL/min

    _____ Hyperactive deep tendon reflexes

    _____ Decreased level of consciousness

    _____ Proteinuria

5. A nurse is collecting data from a client who is pregnant. The client has heart disease and reports fatigue and dyspnea with ordinary exertion. Which of the following is the correct classification for this client's heart disease?

    A. Class I

    B. Class II

    C. Class III

    D. Class IV

APPLICATION EXERCISES ANSWER KEY

1. A nurse is caring for a client at 13 weeks of gestation who is diagnosed with hyperemesis gravidarum. The nurse is aware that which of the following is a risk factor for the client?

    A. Maternal age greater than 40

    B. Vitamin B deficiencies

    C. Oligohydramnios

    D. Placenta previa

    Risk factors for hyperemesis gravidarum include obesity, multifetal gestation, vitamin B deficiencies, and maternal age less than 20. Maternal age greater than 40, oligohydramnios, and placenta previa are not risk factors for clients who have hyperemesis gravidarum.

     NCLEX® Connection: Physiological Adaptation, Alterations in Body Systems

2. A nurse in the antepartum clinic is collecting data for a client who is diagnosed with gestational diabetes mellitus. Which of the following findings indicate hyperglycemia? (Select all that apply.)

    __X__ **Flushed dry skin**

    __X__ **Fruity breath odor**

    __X__ **Hypotension**

    _____ Slurred speech

    _____ Diaphoresis

    Clinical findings for hyperglycemia include flushed dry skin, fruity breath, rapid, weak pulse, and hypotension. Slurred speech and diaphoresis are findings associated with hypoglycemia.

     NCLEX® Connection: Physiological Adaptation, Alterations in Body Systems

3. A nurse is assisting with the care of a client diagnosed with preeclampsia and is prescribed an IV infusion of magnesium sulfate. The nurse is aware that which of the following medications should be available in the event of magnesium sulfate toxicity?

    A. Calcium gluconate

    B. Oxytocin (Pitocin)

    C. Terbutaline (Brethine)

    D. Misoprostol (Cytotec)

    Calcium gluconate is the antidote for magnesium sulfate and will be a standing order to be administered for magnesium sulfate toxicity. Oxytocin and misoprostol are used to induce or augment labor. Terbutaline is used for the treatment of preterm labor.

     NCLEX® Connection: Pharmacological Therapies, Expected Actions/Outcomes

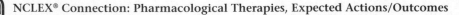

4. A nurse should monitor for which of the following signs of magnesium sulfate toxicity? (Select all that apply.)

X	**Respirations less than 12/min**
X	**Urinary output less than 30 mL/min**
	Hyperactive deep tendon reflexes
X	**Decreased level of consciousness**
	Proteinuria

Signs of magnesium sulfate toxicity include respirations less than 12/min, urine output less than 30 mL/hr, depressed deep tendon reflexes, and a decreased level of consciousness. Proteinuria is a finding of preeclampsia.

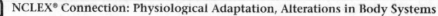 NCLEX® Connection: Physiological Adaptation, Alterations in Body Systems

5. A nurse is collecting data from a client who is pregnant. The client has heart disease and reports fatigue and dyspnea with ordinary exertion. Which of the following is the correct classification for this client's heart disease?

A. Class I

B. Class II

C. Class III

D. Class IV

The classification system will guide the provider in the management of cardiovascular disease. Clients exhibiting clinical findings with ordinary exertion activity are in Class II.

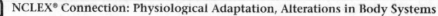 NCLEX® Connection: Physiological Adaptation, Alterations in Body Systems

UNIT 1	ANTEPARTUM NURSING CARE
Section:	Complications of Pregnancy
Chapter 8	Early Onset of Labor

◎ Overview

- Identifying the onset of early labor in clients who are pregnant is crucial for maternal and fetal well-being.

- Preterm labor, premature rupture of membranes, and preterm premature rupture of membranes will be mentioned in this chapter.

PRETERM LABOR

◎ Overview

- Preterm labor is defined as uterine contractions and cervical changes that occur between 20 and 37 weeks of gestation.

Data Collection

- Risk Factors

  - Infections of the urinary tract, vagina, or chorioamnionitis (infection of the amnion)

  - Previous preterm birth

  - Multifetal pregnancy

  - Hydramnios (excessive amniotic fluid)

  - Age below 17 or above 35

  - Low socioeconomic status

  - Smoking, substance abuse

  - Domestic violence

  - History of multiple miscarriages or abortions

  - Diabetes mellitus or hypertension

  - Lack of prenatal care

  - Incompetent cervix

  - Placenta previa or abruptio placentae

- ○ Preterm premature rupture of membranes
- ○ Short interval between pregnancies
- ○ Uterine abnormalities
  - Dehydration – Stimulates the pituitary gland to secrete an antidiuretic hormone and oxytocin. Preventing dehydration will prevent the release of oxytocin, which stimulates uterine contractions.
- Subjective Data
  - ○ Persistent low backache
  - ○ Pressure in the pelvis and cramping
  - ○ Gastrointestinal cramping, sometimes with diarrhea
  - ○ Urinary frequency
  - ○ Vaginal discharge
- Objective Data
  - ○ Physical assessment findings
    - Increase or change in vaginal discharge or bleeding
    - Change in cervical dilation
    - Regular uterine contractions with a frequency of every 10 min or greater, lasting 1 hr or longer
    - Premature rupture of membranes
  - ○ Laboratory tests
    - Vaginal swab for fetal fibronectin, a protein in the amniotic fluid that appears between 24 and 34 weeks of gestation. This protein can be found in the vaginal secretions when the fetal membrane integrity is lost.
    - Cervical cultures
    - CBC, urinalysis
  - ○ Diagnostic procedures
    - Biophysical profile and/or a nonstress test to provide information about the fetal well-being.

Collaborative Care

- Nursing Care
  - ○ Activity restriction
    - Instruct clients to remain on modified bed rest with bathroom privileges.
    - Encourage clients to rest in the left lateral position to increase blood flow to the uterus and decrease uterine activity.

- Tell clients to avoid sexual intercourse.
- Ensure hydration.
  - Encourage clients to consume 2 to 3 L fluids/day from food and beverage sources, preferably milk, water, or juice.
- Identify and treat infection.
  - Have clients report any vaginal discharge, noting color, consistency, and odor.
  - Monitor maternal vital signs.
- Monitor FHR and contraction pattern. Report FHR tachycardia (greater than 160/min).

- Medications
  - Terbutaline (Brethine)
    - Terbutaline is a beta-adrenergic agonist that relaxes uterine smooth muscle by stimulating beta-$_2$ receptors in the smooth muscle fibers to inhibit uterine activity.
    - Nursing considerations
      - Administer orally or by subcutaneous injection.
      - Monitor clients for signs and symptoms of pulmonary edema, which includes chest pain, shortness of breath, respiratory distress, audible wheezing and crackles, and/or a productive cough containing blood-tinged sputum.
        - Monitor the client's daily weights.
        - Restrict the client's oral and IV fluid to 1,500 to 2,400 mL/24 hr to reduce the risk of pulmonary edema.
        - Monitor the client's cardiovascular status. Withhold the client's medication and contact the provider if the maternal heart rate is greater than 120/min.
        - Observe the injection site for infection if administered subcutaneously.
      - Reinforce to clients that medication should be taken around the clock, even through the night. Suggest that clients set an alarm clock to wake up and take it during the night.
    - Client education
      - Reinforce to clients and families about adverse effects to observe for and when to notify the provider.
  - Magnesium sulfate
    - Magnesium sulfate relaxes the smooth muscle of the uterus and thus inhibits uterine activity by suppressing contractions.

- Nursing considerations
  - Assist with the care of clients receiving magnesium sulfate IV.
  - Monitor and report clinical findings of pulmonary edema, which include chest pain, shortness of breath, respiratory distress, audible wheezing and crackles, and/or a productive cough containing blood-tinged sputum.
  - Monitor and report signs of toxicity, which includes loss of deep tendon reflexes, urinary output less than 30 mL/hr, and respiratory rate less than 12/min.
  - Notify the charge nurse of the findings so the medication can be discontinued and the provider notified.
- Client education
  - Instruct clients to report blurred vision, headache, nausea, vomiting, or difficulty breathing.

- Indomethacin (Indocin)
  - Indomethacin is a nonsteroidal anti-inflammatory drug (NSAID) that suppresses preterm labor by blocking the production of prostaglandins. This inhibition of prostaglandins suppresses uterine contractions. Use for gestational age less than 32 weeks.
  - Nursing considerations
    - Monitor clients for dyspepsia, pyrosis, dizziness, oligohydramnios, nausea and vomiting.
    - Monitor clients for postpartum hemorrhage related to reduced platelet aggregation.
    - Administer indomethacin with food or rectally to decrease gastrointestinal distress.
  - Client education
    - Instruct clients to report dizziness, nausea, or vomiting.

- Betamethasone (Celestone)
  - Betamethasone is a glucocorticoid that is administered IM and requires a 24-hr period to be effective. Normally two doses are given 24 hr apart. The therapeutic action is to promote fetal lung maturity and surfactant production.
  - Nursing considerations
    - Administer the medication deep into the client's gluteal muscle.
    - Monitor for pulmonary edema.
    - Monitor for maternal and newborn hyperglycemia.
    - Monitor newborns for changes in heart rate.
  - Client education
    - Instruct clients to report chest pain or shortness of breath.

- Care After Discharge

  o Client education

    ▪ Instruct clients in use of home uterine activity monitoring (HUAM).

- Client Outcomes

  o Client will maintain pregnancy until term.

  o Client's pregnancy will continue to promote fetal lung maturity.

PREMATURE RUPTURE OF MEMBRANES
AND PRETERM PREMATURE RUPTURE OF MEMBRANES

Overview

- Premature rupture of membranes (PROM) is the spontaneous rupture of the amniotic membranes 1 hr or more prior to the onset of true labor. For most women, PROM signifies the onset of true labor if gestational duration is at term.

- Preterm premature rupture of membranes (PPROM) is the premature spontaneous rupture of membranes after 20 weeks of gestation and prior to 37 weeks of gestation.

Data Collection

- Risk Factors

  o Infection is the major risk of PROM and PPROM for both clients and fetuses. Once the amniotic membranes have ruptured, microorganisms can ascend from the vagina into the amniotic sac. PPROM is often preceded by infection.

  o There is an increased risk of infection if delivery takes place greater than 24 hr after the rupture of membranes.

- Subjective Data

  o Reports of a gush or leakage of clear fluid from the vagina.

- Objective Data

  o Physical assessment findings

    ▪ Maternal fever

    ▪ Increased maternal or FHR

    ▪ Foul-smelling fluid or vaginal discharge

    ▪ Visual pool of fluid

    ▪ Abdominal tenderness

    ▪ Prolapsed umbilical cord

    ▪ Abrupt FHR variable or prolonged deceleration

    ▪ Visible or palpable cord at the vaginal introitus

- o Laboratory tests
    - Verify rupture of membranes with positive nitrazine test paper (blue, pH 6.5 to 7.5 indicates a positive test for amniotic fluid), a ferning test (dried fluid on a slide appears in a crystalline pattern under the microscope and indicates the presence of amniotic fluid), or a CBC.
    - Vaginal cultures for streptococcus ß-hemolytic, Group B, Chlamydia, and *Neisseria gonorrhoeae*

Collaborative Care

- Nursing Care
    - o Prepare for birth if indicated.
    - o Provide reassurance to reduce maternal anxiety.
    - o Determine cervical dilation, effacement, and station, but avoid unnecessary vaginal exams.
    - o Check vital signs every 4 hr.
    - o Notify the provider of a temperature greater than 38° C (100° F).
    - o Notify the provider of uterine contractions.
    - o Monitor FHR and uterine contractions.
    - o Maintain clients on bed rest with bathroom privileges.
    - o Encourage hydration.
    - o Obtain vaginal, urine, and blood cultures prior to administration of antibiotic.
- Medications
    - o Ampicillin (Omnipen)
        - Ampicillin is an antibiotic that is used to treat infection.
    - o Betamethasone (Celestone)
        - Betamethasone is a glucocorticoid used to promote lung maturity and surfactant production. It may be administered if chorioamnionitis is not present.
- Care After Discharge
    - o Client education
        - Advise clients to adhere to bed rest with bathroom privileges.
        - Encourage hydration.
        - Instruct clients to:
            - □ Report uterine contractions and foul-smelling vaginal discharge.
            - □ Record daily kick counts for fetal movement.

- □ Abstain from intercourse and avoid tub baths.
- □ Wipe the perineal area from front to back after voiding and fecal elimination.
- Client Outcomes
  - ○ The client will have no presence of fetal or maternal compromise.

(A) APPLICATION EXERCISES

1. A nurse is caring for a client prescribed terbutaline (Brethine) 0.25 mg SQ. Which of the following findings should the nurse report to the provider?

   A. 2+ deep tendon reflex

   B. HR 124

   C. Blood pressure 141/88 mm Hg

   D. 1+ proteinuria

2. A nurse is assisting with the care of a client at 30 weeks of gestation diagnosed with preterm labor. Which of the following medications should the nurse anticipate the provider to prescribe to stop the client's labor? (Select all that apply.)

   _____ Terbutaline (Brethine)

   _____ Indomethacin (Indocin)

   _____ Magnesium Sulfate

   _____ Betamethasone (Celestone)

   _____ Misoprostol (Cytotec)

3. Match the following terms with their appropriate phrase.

   _____ Preterm labor

   _____ Premature rupture of membranes

   _____ Chorioamnionitis

   _____ Preterm premature rupture of membranes

   A. Spontaneous rupture of the amniotic membranes 1 hr or more prior to the onset of true labor

   B. Spontaneous rupture of membranes after 20 weeks gestation and prior to 37 weeks gestation

   C. Infection of the amniotic membranes

   D. Uterine contractions and cervical changes that occur between 20 and 37 weeks gestation

4. A nurse is caring for a client diagnosed with preterm labor. Which of the following are risk factors for this client? (Select all that apply.)

   _____ Oligohydramnios

   _____ Diabetes mellitus

   _____ Chorioamnionitis

   _____ Urinary tract infection

   _____ Smoking

5. A nurse in a clinic is collecting data from a client at 32 weeks of gestation reporting uterine contractions and back discomfort. The nurse is aware that the provider may prescribe which of the following to determine if preterm labor is imminent?

   A. Vaginal swab to check for fetal fibronectin

   B. Biophysical profile

   C. Amniocentesis

   D. Kleihauer-Betke stain

APPLICATION EXERCISES ANSWER KEY

1. A nurse is caring for a client prescribed terbutaline (Brethine) 0.25 mg SQ. Which of the following findings should the nurse report to the provider?

    A. 2+ deep tendon reflex

    B. HR 124

    C. Blood pressure 141/88 mm Hg

    D. 1+ proteinuria

    Maternal heart rate of 120 to 140/min should be reported to the provider and the medication should be withheld. A 2+ deep tendon reflex is within the expected range and does not require notification of the provider. 1+ proteinuria is not an adverse effect of terbutaline. A blood pressure of 141/88 is not an adverse effect of the medication.

    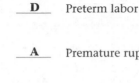 NCLEX® Connection: Physiological Adaptation, Alterations in Body Systems

2. A nurse is assisting with the care of a client at 30 weeks of gestation diagnosed with preterm labor. Which of the following medications should the nurse anticipate the provider to prescribe to stop the client's labor? (Select all that apply.)

__X__	**Terbutaline (Brethine)**
__X__	**Indomethacin (Indocin)**
__X__	**Magnesium Sulfate**
_____	Betamethasone (Celestone)
_____	Misoprostol (Cytotec)

    Terbutaline, Indocin, and Magnesium sulfate are used for the treatment of preterm labor to maintain the pregnancy. Betamethasone may be prescribed if there is no presence of chorioamnionitis. However, it is not used to stop the client's labor. Misoprostol is used as a cervical ripening agent.

    NCLEX® Connection: Physiological Adaptation, Alterations in Body Systems

3. Match the following terms with their appropriate phrase.

__D__	Preterm labor	A. Spontaneous rupture of the amniotic membranes 1 hr or more prior to the onset of true labor
__A__	Premature rupture of membranes	B. Spontaneous rupture of membranes after 20 weeks gestation and prior to 37 weeks gestation
__C__	Chorioamnionitis	C. Infection of the amniotic membranes
__B__	Preterm premature rupture of membranes	D. Uterine contractions and cervical changes that occur between 20 and 37 weeks gestation

    NCLEX® Connection: Physiological Adaptation, Alterations in Body Systems

4. A nurse is caring for a client diagnosed with preterm labor. Which of the following are risk factors for this client? (Select all that apply.)

_____ Oligohydramnios

__X__ **Diabetes mellitus**

__X__ **Chorioamnionitis**

__X__ **Urinary tract infection**

__X__ **Smoking**

Smoking, diabetes mellitus, chorioamnionitis, hydramnios, and urinary tract infections are risk factors for the development of preterm labor. Oligohydramnios is not a risk factor.

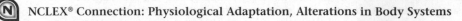 NCLEX® Connection: Physiological Adaptation, Alterations in Body Systems

5. A nurse in a clinic is collecting data from a client at 32 weeks of gestation reporting uterine contractions and back discomfort. The nurse is aware that the provider may prescribe which of the following to determine if preterm labor is imminent?

A. Vaginal swab to check for fetal fibronectin

B. Biophysical profile

C. Amniocentesis

D. Kleihauer-Betke stain

A vaginal swab for fetal fibronectin may be prescribed between 24 and 34 weeks of gestation to determine if the client might experience preterm labor. Biophysical profile is used to evaluate fetal well-being. An amniocentesis is used to determine fetal lung maturity. A Kleihauer-Betke stain is used to detect for the presence of a transplacental hemorrhage.

NCLEX® Connection: Physiological Adaptation, Alterations in Body Systems

UNIT 2: INTRAPARTUM NURSING CARE

- Nursing Care of the Client in Labor
- Fetal Assessment During Labor

NCLEX® CONNECTIONS

When reviewing the chapters in this section, keep in mind the relevant sections of the NCLEX® outline, in particular:

CLIENT NEEDS: HEALTH PROMOTION AND MAINTENANCE	CLIENT NEEDS: PHARMACOLOGICAL THERAPIES	CLIENT NEEDS: PHYSIOLOGICAL ADAPTATION

Relevant topics/tasks include:
 	
- Ante/Intra/Postpartum and Newborn Care
  - Assist with monitoring a client in labor.
- Data Collection Techniques
  - Collect baseline physical data.
	Relevant topics/tasks include:
	
	- Adverse Effects/ Contraindications/Side Effects/Interactions
	  - Identify a contraindication to the administration of prescribed over-the-counter medication to the client.
	- Dosage Calculation
	  - Use clinical decision making/critical thinking when calculating dosages.
	- Pharmacological Pain Management
	  - Monitor client non-verbal signs of pain/ discomfort.
		Relevant topics/tasks include:
		
		- Alterations in Body Systems
		  - Provide care for a client experiencing complications of pregnancy/labor and/ or delivery.
		- Medical Emergencies
		  - Notify primary health care provider about client unexpected response/emergency situation.

UNIT 2	INTRAPARTUM NURSING CARE
Chapter 9	Nursing Care of the Client in Labor

◎ Overview

- Intrapartum nursing care involves caring for clients just prior to the onset of labor, during the labor process, and the immediate period after delivery of the newborn.

- The labor and birth process starts when clients experience the physiological changes that precede labor or when the process is initiated by the provider. Care may include use of a Bishop score, cervical ripening, induction/augmentation of labor, monitoring of FHR and uterine contractions, and pain management. Clients will present to a health care facility to begin the labor process and will be discharged after the delivery of the newborn in the early postpartum period.

Cervical Ripening, Labor Induction, Labor Augmentation

- Cervical ripening increases cervical readiness for labor by either a chemical or mechanical method to promote cervical softening, dilation, and effacement.

  ○ Chemical agents consist of prostaglandin E_1 (misoprostol [Cytotec] and prostaglandin E_2, dinoprostone [Cervidil Insert]), which is used to "ripen" the cervix (soften and thin) and to increase cervical readiness prior to the induction of labor.

- Induction of labor is the deliberate initiation of uterine contractions to stimulate labor before spontaneous onset to bring about the birth either by chemical or mechanical means.

- Augmentation of labor is the stimulation of hypotonic contractions once labor has spontaneously begun, but progress is inadequate.

- Methods

  ○ Amniotomy or stripping of membranes

  ○ Prostaglandins applied cervically

  ○ Nipple stimulation to trigger the release of endogenous oxytocin

  ○ Administration of IV oxytocin (Pitocin)

- Indications

  ○ Diagnoses

    ▪ Any condition in which augmentation or induction of labor is indicated

- Client Outcomes

  o The client's labor will progress without complications.

- Nursing Actions

  o Preparation of Client

    ▪ Determine Bishop score to evaluate maternal readiness for labor.

    ▪ Assign a numerical value of 0 to 3 for cervical dilation, cervical effacement, cervical consistency, cervical position, and presenting part station.

      □ A score of 9 for nulliparas and 5 or more for multiparas indicates readiness for labor induction.

    ▪ Obtain the client's consent.

    ▪ Obtain baseline FHR, maternal vital signs, and contraction pattern.

- Ongoing Care

  o Prepare clients for an amniotomy or amniotic membrane stripping.

  o Assist with the care of clients receiving cervical-ripening agents, undergoing amniotomy or amniotic membrane stripping, or oxytocin (Pitocin) IV infusion.

  o Continue to monitor FHR and uterine activity.

Monitoring Clients During Labor

- Electronic fetal monitoring is a tool to evaluate FHR patterns. First, perform Leopold's maneuvers. Then, assist clients to a semi-sitting or lateral position. Apply conductive gel to an external ultrasound transducer and place on the client's abdomen to monitor the FHR. Place a tocotransducer over the fundus to measure uterine frequency, duration, and regularity.

- Indications

  o Diagnoses

    ▪ Term delivery

  o Client presentation

    ▪ Premonitory Signs of Labor

      □ Backache – A constant low, dull backache, caused by pelvic muscle relaxation

      □ Weight loss – A 0.5 to 1 kg (1 to 3 lb) weight loss

      □ Lightening – Fetal head descends into true pelvis about 14 days before labor; feeling that the fetus has "dropped;" easier breathing, but more pressure on bladder, resulting in urinary frequency; more pronounced in clients who are primigravida

      □ Contractions – Begin with irregular uterine contractions (Braxton Hicks) that eventually progress in strength and regularity

☐ Bloody show – Brownish or blood-tinged mucus discharge caused by expulsion of the cervical mucus plug resulting from the onset of cervical dilation and effacement

☐ Energy burst – Sometimes called "nesting" response

☐ Gastrointestinal changes – Less common, include nausea, vomiting, and indigestion

☐ Rupture of membranes – Spontaneous rupture of membranes can initiate labor or occur anytime during labor, most commonly during the transition phase.

☐ Labor usually occurs within 24 hr of the rupture of membranes.

☐ Prolonged rupture of membranes greater than 24 hr before delivery of fetus may lead to an infection.

- Client Outcomes

  o The client will progress through the labor process without complications.

  o The client will deliver a newborn without complications

- Preprocedure

  o Nursing actions

    ▪ Perform initial data collection for admission to the birthing facility.

      ☐ Provide culturally competent care that respects and is compatible with the client's culture.

      ☐ Conduct an admission history, review of antepartum care, and review of the birth plan.

      ☐ Obtain laboratory results.

      ☐ Monitor baseline fetal heart tones and uterine contraction patterns for 20 to 30 min.

      ☐ Obtain maternal vital signs.

    ▪ Check the status of the amniotic membranes. Check FHR pattern immediately following the rupture of membranes. Changes in FHR pattern may indicate prolapsed umbilical cord. Note abrupt decelerations and report to provider.

    ▪ Observer amniotic fluid

      ☐ Color should be pale to straw yellow

      ☐ Odor should not be foul

      ☐ Clarity should appear watery and clear

      ☐ Volume is between 500 to 1,200 mL

      ☐ Use nitrazine paper to test fluid to confirm that it is amniotic.

        ▸ Nitrazine tests the pH of the amniotic fluid. Deep blue (6.5 to 7.5) indicates fluid that is alkaline. If the fluid strip is yellow, this indicates slight acidity because the fluid is urine.

■ Determine if client is in true labor.

CHARACTERISTICS OF TRUE VS. FALSE LABOR (BRAXTON HICKS CONTRACTIONS)	
TRUE LABOR	**FALSE LABOR**

• Contractions
  ○ May begin irregularly, but become regular in frequency
  ○ Stronger, last longer, and are more frequent
  ○ Felt in lower back, radiating to abdomen
  ○ Walking can increase contraction intensity
  ○ Continue despite comfort measures
	• Contractions
	  ○ Painless, irregular frequency, and intermittent
	  ○ Decrease in frequency, duration, and intensity with walking or position changes
	  ○ Felt in lower back or abdomen above umbilicus
	  ○ Often stop with sleep or comfort measures such as oral hydration or emptying of the bladder

• Cervix (assessed by vaginal exam)
  ○ Progressive change in dilation and effacement
  ○ Moves to anterior position
  ○ Bloody show
	• Cervix (assessed by vaginal exam)
	  ○ No significant change in dilation or effacement
	  ○ Often remains in posterior position
	  ○ No significant bloody show

• Fetus
  ○ Presenting part engages in pelvis
	• Fetus
	  ○ Presenting part is not engaged in pelvis

■ Obtain clean-catch urine samples for urinalysis to ascertain maternal:

    □ Hydration status via specific gravity.

    □ Nutritional status via ketones.

    □ Proteinuria, which is indicative of preeclampsia.

    □ Urinary tract infection via bacterial count.

    □ Beta-strep culture to check for streptococcus ß-hemolytic, Group B.

■ Review blood tests

    □ Hct level

    □ ABO typing and Rh-factor if not previously done

○ Client education

■ Provide clients and families with ongoing education regarding the labor and delivery process and procedures.

• Intraprocedure

■ Nursing actions

    □ Perform Leopold's maneuvers.

- □ Check maternal vital signs per facility protocol.

- □ Check maternal temperature every 1 to 2 hr if membranes are ruptured.

- □ Apply external monitoring equipment.

- □ Apply the tocodynamometer (tocotransducer) to the client's abdomen over the fundus to measure uterine activity.

 View Media Supplement: Contraction Pattern (Animation)

  - ▸ Duration – the time between the beginning of a contraction to the end of that same contraction. Duration greater than 90 seconds may cause a decrease in fetal oxygenation.

  - ▸ Intensity – strength of the contraction at its peak described as mild, moderate, or strong.

  - ▸ Frequency – time from beginning of one contraction to the beginning of the next contraction. Interval between contractions should not be less than 60 seconds to maintain fetal oxygenation.

  - ▸ Resting tone of uterine contractions – tone of the uterine muscle in between contractions.

- □ Apply the ultrasound transducer (external fetal monitoring (EFM) transducer) to the client's abdomen to monitor FHR patterns.

- □ Encourage clients to void every 2 hr to prevent bladder distention.

- □ Encourage clients to change positions frequently.

- □ Assist with a vaginal examination – Performed digitally by the provider or qualified nurse to assess for:

  - ▸ Cervical dilation (stretching of cervical os adequate to allow fetal passage) and effacement (cervical thinning and shortening)

  - ▸ Descent of the fetus through the birth canal as measured by fetal station in centimeters

  - ▸ Fetal position, presenting part, and lie

- □ Assist with monitoring clients in labor.

STAGES OF LABOR			
STAGE	BEGINS WITH	ENDS WITH	MATERNAL CHARACTERISTICS
First stage: 12 1/2 hr (average)	• Onset of labor	• Complete dilation	• Cervical dilation 1 cm/hr for clients who are primigravida, and 1.5 cm/hr for clients who are multigravida, on average

Latent Phase:
• Duration Primigravida:
  o 6 hr (approximately)
• Duration Multigravida:
  o 4 hr (approximately)
	• Cervix 0 cm
	• Irregular, mild to moderate contractions
	• Frequency 5 to 30 min
	• Duration 30 to 45 seconds
		• Cervix 3 cm	• Some dilation and effacement
			• Talkative and eager

Active Phase:
• Duration Primigravida:
  o 3 hr (approximately)
• Duration Multigravida:
  o 2 hr (approximately)
	• Cervix 4 cm
	• More regular, moderate to strong contractions
	• Frequency 3 to 5 min
	• Duration 40 to 70 seconds
		• Cervix 7 cm dilated	• Rapid dilation and effacement
			• Some fetal descent
			• Feelings of helplessness
			• Anxiety and restlessness, introverted, increase as contractions become stronger

Transition: • Duration: o Approximately 20 to 40 min	• Cervix 8 cm • Strong to very strong contractions • Frequency 2 to 3 min • Duration 45 to 90 seconds	• Complete dilation at 10 cm	• Tired, restless, and irritable • Feeling out of control, client often states, "cannot continue" • May have nausea and vomiting • Urge to push • Increased rectal pressure and feelings of needing to have a bowel movement • Increased bloody show • Most difficult part of labor

STAGES OF LABOR			
STAGE	BEGINS WITH	ENDS WITH	MATERNAL CHARACTERISTICS

Second Stage:
• Duration Primigravida:
  ○ 30 min to 2 hr
• Duration Multigravida:
  ○ 5 to 30 min
	• Full dilation
	• Intense contractions every 1 to 2 min
		• Birth	• Pushing results in birth of fetus

Third Stage: • Duration Primigravida and Multigravida: ○ 5 to 30 min	• Delivery of the newborn	• Delivery of placenta	• Placental separation and expulsion • Schultze presentation: shiny fetal surface of placenta emerges first • Duncan presentation: dull maternal surface of placenta emerges first
Fourth Stage: • Duration Primigravida and Multigravida: ○ 1 to 4 hr	• Delivery of placenta	• Maternal stabilization of vital signs	• Achievement of vital sign homeostasis • Lochia scant to moderate rubra

View Media Supplement:

• Stages of Labor (Video) • Schultze and Dirty Duncan Placenta (Images)

    ☐   Discourage pushing efforts until the cervix is fully dilated.

    ☐   Observe for perineal bulging or crowning (appearance of the fetal head at the perineum).

    ☐   Encourage clients to begin bearing down with contractions once the cervix is fully dilated. Listen for client statements expressing the need to have a bowel movement. This sensation is a sign of complete dilation and fetal descent.

    ☐   Assist with providing pain management

TIMING AND EFFECTIVENESS OF PAIN RELIEF MEASURES DURING LABOR				
First Stage (Latent Phase)	First Stage (Active Phase)	Transition	Second Stage	Third Stage
Nonpharmacological methods ⟶				
Sedatives			Spinal Block ⟶	
	Opioids			
	Epidural ⟶			
			Pudendal ⟶	
			Local infiltration ⟶	

Nonpharmacological Pain Management

- Assist clients to use nonpharmacological measures to promote relaxation and relieve the discomfort of labor. These include breathing techniques, effleurage, music, massage, sacral counterpressure, hydrotherapy, and heat or cold therapy.

- Indications

    o Diagnosis

      ■ Term delivery

    o Client presentation

      ■ Client reports pain.

    o Client outcomes

      ■ The client effectively promotes relaxation and manages pain during labor.

      ■ The client reports relief of labor discomforts.

    o Nursing actions

      ■ Assist clients with breathing techniques. Encourage deep cleansing breaths. Check for signs of hyperventilation (caused by low blood levels of PCO_2 from blowing off too much CO_2) such as light-headedness and tingling of the fingers.

        □ If hyperventilation occurs, have clients breathe into a paper bag or her cupped hands.

      ■ Assist clients with sensory stimulation strategies to promote relaxation and pain relief:

        □ Aroma therapy

        □ Breathing techniques

        □ Imagery

        □ Music

        □ Use of focal points

- Assist clients with cutaneous strategies to promote relaxation and pain relief:
  - Back rubs and massage
  - Effleurage
    - Light, gentle circular stroking of the client's abdomen with the fingertips in rhythm with breathing during contractions
  - Sacral counterpressure
    - Consistent pressure is applied by the support person using the heel of the hand or fist against the client's sacral area to counteract pain in the lower back.
  - Heat or cold therapy
  - Hydrotherapy (whirlpool or shower) increases maternal endorphin levels
  - Intradermal water block
  - Hypnosis
  - Acupressure
    - Transcutaneous electrical nerve stimulation (TENS) unit
- Promote frequent maternal position changes to promote relaxation and pain relief:
  - Semi-sitting
  - Squatting
  - Kneeling
  - Kneeling and rocking back and forth
  - Supine position only with the placement of a wedge under one of the client's hips to tilt the uterus and avoid supine hypotension syndrome

Pharmacological Pain Management

- Alleviates pain sensations or raises the threshold for pain perception

- Clients may be given IM or IV opioid analgesics as a pharmacological method of pain management. Epidural and spinal regional analgesia may be administered by an anesthesia care provider. Regional blocks, such as a pudendal block or, a paracervical nerve block, may be administered by the provider to provide local anesthesia to the perineum, vulva, and rectal areas during delivery, episiotomy, and episiotomy repair.

- Indications
  - Diagnosis
    - Term delivery
  - Client presentation
    - The client reports pain.

- o Client outcomes
  - Clients report relief of labor pain and discomforts
- o Nursing actions
  - Opioid analgesics such as meperidine hydrochloride (Demerol), fentanyl (Sublimaze), butorphanol (Stadol), and nalbuphine (Nubain) act in the CNS to decrease the perception of pain without the loss of consciousness. Clients may be given opioid analgesics IM or IV, but the IV route is recommended during labor because action is quicker.
    - □ Butorphanol (Stadol) and nalbuphine (Nubain) provide pain relief without causing significant respiratory depression in the mother or fetus.
  - Monitor clients for adverse effects
    - □ Crosses the placental barrier; if given to the mother too close to the time of delivery, can cause respiratory depression in the newborn.
    - □ Reduces gastric emptying; increases the risk for nausea and emesis
    - □ Increases the risk for aspiration of food or fluids in the stomach
    - □ Sedation
    - □ Tachycardia
    - □ Hypotension
    - □ Decreased FHR variability
    - □ Allergic reaction
  - Have naloxone (Narcan) available to counteract the effects of respiratory depression in the newborn.
    - □ Administer antiemetics as prescribed.
    - □ Monitor maternal vital signs, uterine contraction pattern, and FHR.
    - □ Dim the lights and provide a quiet atmosphere.
    - □ Provide safety for the client by lowering the position of the bed and elevate the side rails.
- o Client education
  - Explain to clients that the medication will cause drowsiness.
  - Instruct clients to request assistance with ambulation.
  - Phenothiazine medications such as promethazine (Phenergan) or hydroxyzine (Vistaril) can control nausea and anxiety. They do not relieve pain and are used as an adjunct with opioids.
- o Nursing actions
  - Monitor for sedation and dry mouth
    - □ Provide ice chips or mouth swabs.
    - □ Provide safety measures to clients.

- ○ Epidural and spinal regional analgesia consists of using analgesics such as fentanyl (Sublimaze) and sufentanil (Sufenta), which are short-acting opioids that are administered as a motor block into the epidural or intrathecal space without anesthesia. These opioids produce regional analgesia, providing rapid pain relief while still allowing clients to sense contractions and maintain the ability to bear down.

- ○ Nursing actions

  - ▪ Monitor clients for adverse effects

    - ☐ Decreased gastric emptying resulting in nausea and vomiting

    - ☐ Inhibition of bowel and bladder elimination sensations

    - ☐ Bradycardia or tachycardia

    - ☐ Hypotension

    - ☐ Respiratory depression

    - ☐ Allergic reaction and pruritus

  - ▪ Institute safety precautions, such as putting side rails up on the client's bed. Clients may experience dizziness and sedation, which increases maternal risk for injury.

  - ▪ Monitor clients for nausea and emesis and administer antiemetics as prescribed.

  - ▪ Monitor maternal vital signs per facility protocol.

  - ▪ Monitor for allergic reaction.

  - ▪ Continue FHR pattern monitoring.

- ○ Client education

  - ▪ Provide clients with ongoing education related to expectations for procedure.

- ○ Anesthesia used in childbirth includes regional blocks and general anesthesia (rarely used).

- ○ Regional blocks are most commonly used and consist of pudendal block, epidural block, spinal block, and paracervical nerve block. Pharmacological anesthesia eliminates pain perceptions by interrupting the nerve impulses to the brain.

  - ▪ Pudendal block consists of a local anesthetic such as lidocaine (Xylocaine) or bupivacaine (Marcaine) being administered transvaginally into the space in front of the pudendal nerve. This type of block has no maternal or fetal systemic effects, but it does provide local anesthesia to the perineum, vulva, and rectal areas during delivery, episiotomy, and episiotomy repair. It is administered during the second stage of labor 10 to 20 min before delivery providing analgesia prior to spontaneous expulsion of the fetus or forceps-assisted or vacuum-assisted birth.

- ○ Nursing actions

  - ▪ Monitor clients for adverse effects.

  - ▪ Broad ligament hematoma

- Compromise of maternal bearing-down reflex
- Coach clients about when to bear down.
- Check the perineal and vulvar area postpartum for hematoma.
  - ○ Client education
    - Provide clients with ongoing education related to expectations for procedure
  - ○ An epidural block consists of a local anesthetic bupivacaine (Marcaine) along with an analgesic morphine (Duramorph) or fentanyl (Sublimaze) injected into the epidural space at the level of the fourth or fifth vertebrae. This eliminates all sensation from the level of the umbilicus to the thighs, relieving the discomfort of uterine contractions, fetal descent, and pressure and stretching of the perineum. It is administered when clients are in active labor and dilated to at least 4 cm. Continuous infusion or intermittent injections may be administered through an indwelling epidural catheter. Patient-controlled epidural analgesia is a new technique for labor analgesia and is becoming a favored method of acute pain relief management for labor and birth.
  - ○ Nursing actions
    - Monitor clients for adverse effects
    - Maternal hypotension
    - Fetal bradycardia
    - Inability to feel the urge to void
    - Loss of the bearing-down reflex
    - Monitor clients receiving a bolus of IV fluids to help offset maternal hypotension as prescribed.
    - Help to position and steady clients into either a sitting or side-lying modified Sims' position, with client's back curved to widen the intervertebral space for insertion of the epidural catheter.
    - Encourage clients to remain in the side-lying position after insertion of the epidural catheter to avoid supine hypotension syndrome with compression of the vena cava.
    - Coach clients in pushing efforts and request an evaluation of epidural pain management by anesthesia if pushing efforts are ineffective.
    - Monitor maternal blood pressure and pulse, observe for hypotension, respiratory depression, and oxygen saturations.
    - Monitor FHR patterns continuously.
    - Ensure oxygen and suction equipment is available.
    - Provide client safety such as raising the side rails of the bed. Do not allow clients to ambulate unassisted until all motor control has returned.
    - Check the maternal bladder for distention at frequent intervals and catheterize if necessary to assist with voiding.
    - Monitor for the return of sensation in the client's legs after delivery but prior to standing. Assist clients with standing and walking for the first time after a delivery that included epidural anesthesia.

- ○ Client education
  - ▪ Provide ongoing instructions related to the procedure and nursing actions.
- ○ Spinal block consists of a local anesthetic that is injected into the subarachnoid space into the spinal fluid at the third, fourth, or fifth lumbar interspace. This can be done alone or in combination with an analgesic such as fentanyl (Sublimaze). The spinal block eliminates all sensations from the level of the nipples to the feet. It is commonly used for cesarean births. A low spinal block may be used for a vaginal birth, but is not used for labor. A spinal block is administered in the late second stage or before cesarean birth.
- ○ Nursing actions
  - ▪ Monitor clients for adverse effects
    - ▫ Maternal hypotension
    - ▫ Fetal bradycardia
    - ▫ Loss of the bearing-down reflex in the mother with a higher incidence of operative births
    - ▫ Potential headache from leakage of cerebrospinal fluid at the puncture site
    - ▫ Bladder and uterine atony following birth
    - ▫ Check maternal vital signs per facility protocol.
    - ▫ Monitor FHR patterns continuously.
    - ▫ Provide client safety to prevent injury by raising the side rails of the bed and assisting clients with repositioning and ambulating.
    - ▫ Encourage interventions to relieve a postpartum headache resulting from a cerebrospinal fluid leak. Interventions include placing clients in a supine position, promoting bed rest in a dark room, administering oral analgesics, caffeine, and fluids. An autologous blood patch is the most beneficial and reliable relief measure for cerebrospinal fluid leaks.
- ○ Client education
  - ▪ Instruct clients about the method.
- ● Postprocedure
  - ○ Nursing actions
    - ▪ Check maternal vital signs every 15 min for the first hour and then according to facility protocol.
    - ▪ Check fundus and lochia every 15 min for the first hour and then according to facility protocol.
    - ▪ Massage the uterine fundus and/or administer oxytocics as prescribed to maintain uterine tone and to prevent hemorrhage.
    - ▪ Encourage voiding to prevent bladder distention.
    - ▪ Promote an opportunity for maternal-infant bonding.

- Complications

  o Fetal distress

    ■ Indications include:

      □ The FHR is below 110/min or above 160/min.

      □ The FHR shows decreased or no variability.

      □ There is fetal hyperactivity or no fetal activity.

      □ The fetal blood pH is less than 7.2.

  o Nursing actions

      □ Notify the provider.

      □ Assist the chargenurse to:

        ▸ Position clients in a side-lying reclining position with legs elevated to increase uteroplacental perfusion.

        ▸ Administer 8 to 10 L/min of oxygen via a face mask.

        ▸ Maintain IV infusion at 200 mL/min or as prescribed.

        ▸ Prepare clients for an emergency cesarean birth.

  o Client education

      ■ Provide support to clients and their families

- Prolapsed cord

  o A prolapsed umbilical cord occurs when the umbilical cord is displaced, preceding the presenting part of the fetus, or protruding through the cervix. Visualization or palpation of the umbilical cord protruding from the introitus results in cord compression and compromised fetal circulation. Extreme increase in fetal activity that occurs and then ceases is suggestive of severe fetal hypoxia. Risk factors include transverse lie, multifetal pregnancy, cephalopelvic disproportion, an unusually long umbilical cord, and polyhydramnios.

  o Nursing actions

      ■ Call for assistance immediately.

      ■ Have another nurse notify MD immediately.

      ■ Use a sterile-gloved hand, insert two fingers into the vagina, and apply finger pressure on either side of the cord to the fetal presenting part to elevate it off of the cord.

      ■ Place rolled towel under the client's right or left hip to relieve pressure on the cord.

      ■ Reposition clients in a knee-chest, Trendelenburg, or a side-lying position.

      ■ Apply a sterile, saline-soaked towel to the cord to prevent drying and to maintain blood flow if it is protruding from the vaginal introitus.

- Assist the charge nurse to:
  - Monitor the FHR.
  - Administer oxygen at 8 to 10 L/min via a face mask. This will improve fetal oxygenation.
  - Initiate IV infusion or administer a bolus.
  - Prepare clients for a cesarean birth.
- Client education
  - Provide support to clients and their families.

Ⓐ APPLICATION EXERCISES

1. A client reports that her contractions started about 1 hr ago and decreased after drinking two glasses of water and walking. She reports the contractions occur every 10 to 15 min and that she hasn't had any fluid leaking or vaginal bleeding. The nurse should recognize that the client is experiencing

    A. Braxton Hicks contractions.

    B. rupture of membranes.

    C. fetal descent.

    D. true contractions.

2. Identify and describe the three phases of the first stage of labor.

3. While assisting the nurse with an admission history for a client at 39 weeks of gestation, the client tells the nurse that water has been leaking from her vagina for 2 days. The nurse knows that this client is at risk for

    A. cord prolapse.

    B. infection.

    C. postpartum hemorrhage.

    D. hydramnios.

4. A nurse is reinforcing nonpharmacologic pain interventions for lower back pain due to occiput posterior presentation with a group of clients. Which of the following statements regarding nonpharmacologic interventions indicates the client understands an effective intervention for this type of pain?

    A. "I should use effleurage to alleviate the discomfort."

    B. "I will get my husband to apply sacral counterpressure during labor."

    C. "I will try hydrotherapy during my labor to relieve the back pain."

    D. "I should use massage throughout my labor."

5. A nurse is assisting with the care of a primipara in active labor who received meperidine (Demerol) 50 mg IV bolus for pain 30 min prior to precipitous delivery. The nurse is aware that naloxone (Narcan) is to be administered to the newborn for which of the following?

    A. Hypoglycemia

    B. Hyperbilirubinemia

    C. Respiratory depression

    D. Maternal substance abuse

6. A nurse is assisting with the management of a client who is in active labor. Which of the following findings should the nurse report following epidural placement?

    A. Blood pressure 89/54
    B. 2+ pedal edema
    C. Early decelerations
    D. Fetal heart rate 160

7. A nurse is assisting with the care of a client in labor undergoing an induction with oxytocin (Pitocin) by IV infusion. Fetal distress is noted by fetal bradycardia. Which of the following nursing actions should the nurse assist with? (Select all that apply.)

    _____   Place the client in side lying position.
    _____   Maintain primary IV infusion at 200 mL/hr.
    _____   Administer oxygen 8 to 10 mL/min via face mask.
    _____   Administer naloxone (Narcan).
    _____   Increase the rate of oxytocin infusion.

8. A nurse is collecting data from a client in labor following epidural placement. Which of the following findings are adverse effects from the epidural?

    A. Pruritus
    B. Hypertension
    C. Urinary frequency
    D. Maternal temperature

9. A nurse is assisting with the care of a client in labor. The nurse is aware that which of the following are risk factors for umbilical cord prolapse? (Select all that apply.)

    _____   Oligohydramnios
    _____   Transverse lie
    _____   Multifetal pregnancy
    _____   Short umbilical cord
    _____   Cephalopelvic disproportion

APPLICATION EXERCISES ANSWER KEY

1. A client reports that her contractions started about 1 hr ago and decreased after drinking two glasses of water and walking. She reports the contractions occur every 10 to 15 min and that she hasn't had any fluid leaking or vaginal bleeding. The nurse should recognize that the client is experiencing

   A. Braxton Hicks contractions.

   B. rupture of membranes.

   C. fetal descent.

   D. true contractions.

   Braxton Hicks contractions decrease with hydration and walking. True contractions do not go away with hydration or walking. Instead, they are regular in frequency, duration, and intensity, becoming stronger with walking. Fetal descent is the downward movement of the fetus in the birth canal. Rupture of membranes is when the amniotic membranes rupture and allow the amniotic fluid to escape.

   NCLEX® Connection: Health Promotion and Maintenance, Ante/Intra/Postpartum and Newborn Care

2. Identify and describe the three phases of the first stage of labor.

   In stage 1, latent phase, the cervix dilates from 0 to 3 cm, and contraction duration ranges from 30 to 45 sec. In stage 1, active phase, the cervix dilates from 4 to 7 cm, and contraction duration ranges from 40 to 70 sec. In stage 1, transition phase, the cervix dilates from 8 to 10 cm, and contraction duration ranges from 45 to 90 sec.

   NCLEX® Connection: Health Promotion and Maintenance, Ante/Intra/Postpartum and Newborn Care

3. While assisting the nurse with an admission history for a client at 39 weeks of gestation, the client tells the nurse that water has been leaking from her vagina for 2 days. The nurse knows that this client is at risk for

   A. cord prolapse.

   B. infection.

   C. postpartum hemorrhage.

   D. hydramnios.

   Rupture of membranes exceeding 24 hr before delivery increases the risk of infectious organisms entering vaginally into the uterus. While cord prolapse is a risk with rupture of membranes, it occurs when the fluid rushes out rather than trickling or leaking out. The client is not at any greater risk than other pregnant clients for postpartum hemorrhage. Hydramnios means excess amniotic fluid. The client is more likely to have oligohydramnios or insufficient amniotic fluid.

   NCLEX® Connection: Physiological Adaptation, Alterations in Body Systems

4. A nurse is reinforcing nonpharmacologic pain interventions for lower back pain due to occiput posterior presentation with a group of clients. Which of the following statements regarding nonpharmacologic interventions indicates the client understands an effective intervention for this type of pain?

 A. "I should use effleurage to alleviate the discomfort."

 B. "I will get my husband to apply sacral counterpressure during labor."

 C. "I will try hydrotherapy during my labor to relieve the back pain."

 D. "I should use massage throughout my labor."

 Sacral counterpressure is the application of steady pressure to the lower back to counteract the pressure exerted on the spinal nerves by the fetus, which especially occurs with an occiput posterior presentation. Abdominal effleurage is a gentle stroking of the abdomen in rhythm with breathing during contractions. Hydrotherapy may be helpful, but counterpressure is the most effective in relieving back discomfort.

(N) NCLEX® Connection: Basic Care and Comfort, Complementary and Alternative Therapies

5. A nurse is assisting with the care of a primipara in active labor who received meperidine (Demerol) 50 mg IV bolus for pain 30 min prior to precipitous delivery. The nurse is aware that naloxone (Narcan) is to be administered to the newborn for which of the following?

 A. Hypoglycemia

 B. Hyperbilirubinemia

 C. Respiratory depression

 D. Maternal substance abuse

 Naloxone (Narcan) is an opioid antagonist that should be administered to the newborn for respiratory depression. Hypoglycemia, hyperbilirubinemia, and maternal substance abuse are not indications for naloxone administration.

(N) NCLEX® Connection: Pharmacological Therapies, Pharmacological Pain Management

6. A nurse is assisting with the management of a client who is in active labor. Which of the following findings should the nurse report following epidural placement?

 A. Blood pressure 89/54

 B. 2+ pedal edema

 C. Early decelerations

 D. Fetal heart rate 160

 Monitor the mother for hypotension as it is an adverse effect of epidural analgesia. Epidurals have no effect on maternal edema. The fetal heart rate of 160 is within the expected range and early decelerations are common as labor processes.

(N) NCLEX® Connection: Pharmacological Therapies, Parenteral/Intravenous Therapy

7. A nurse is assisting with the care of a client in labor undergoing an induction with oxytocin (Pitocin) by IV infusion. Fetal distress is noted by fetal bradycardia. Which of the following nursing actions should the nurse assist with? (Select all that apply.)

__X__   **Place the client in side lying position.**

__X__   **Maintain primary IV infusion at 200 mL/hr.**

__X__   **Administer oxygen 8 to 10 mL/min via face mask.**

_____   Administer naloxone (Narcan).

_____   Increase the rate of oxytocin infusion.

The nurse should assist with positioning the client laterally, increasing IV fluids, and administering oxygen. There is no indication to administer naloxone, which is an opioid antagonist and is used to correct neonatal depression caused by maternal opioids. The rate of the oxytocin infusion should not be increased, as this may lead to further fetal distress by increasing the rate and intensity of uterine contractions.

 NCLEX® Connection: Health Promotion and Maintenance, Ante/Intra/Postpartum and Newborn Care

8. A nurse is collecting data from a client in labor following epidural placement. Which of the following findings are adverse effects from the epidural?

A. Pruritus

B. Hypertension

C. Urinary frequency

D. Maternal temperature

Pruritus is an adverse effect that the client may experience following the placement of an epidural. Hypertension, urinary frequency, and maternal temperature are not adverse effects.

 NCLEX® Connection: Pharmacological Therapies, Adverse Effects/Contraindications/Side Effects/Interactions

9. A nurse is assisting with the care of a client in labor. The nurse is aware that which of the following are risk factors for umbilical cord prolapse? (Select all that apply.)

__X__   **Oligohydramnios**

__X__   **Transverse lie**

__X__   **Multifetal pregnancy**

_____   Short umbilical cord

__X__   **Cephalopelvic disproportion**

Risk factors for umbilical cord prolapse include transverse lie, multifetal pregnancy, cephalopelvic disproportion, an unusually long umbilical cord, and polyhydramnios. Oligohydramnios and a short umbilical cord are not risk factors.

NCLEX® Connection: Physiological Adaptation, Alterations in Body Systems

UNIT 2	INTRAPARTUM NURSING CARE
Chapter 10	Fetal Assessment During Labor

Overview

- Describe fetal assessment during labor.

- The diagnostic procedures mentioned in this chapter include FHR pattern and uterine contraction monitoring, Leopold's maneuvers, fetal scalp blood sampling, and fetal oxygen monitoring.

LEOPOLD'S MANEUVERS

- Description of Procedure

  - Leopold's maneuvers consist of performing external palpations of the maternal uterus through the abdominal wall:

- Indications

  - To determine:

    - Number of fetuses – One, two, or more fetuses

    - Presenting part – Cephalic, breech, or shoulder

    - Fetal attitude – The posture of the fetus in the uterus. Usually, the fetus is in a posture of general flexion with the chin, hips, and legs flexed inward toward the body, and the arms are crossed with the umbilical lying between the arms and the legs.

    - Fetal lie – Longitudinal or transverse.

    - Fetal position – How the presenting part is positioned in the maternal pelvis in relation to the four quadrants of the pelvis.

    - Station – The degree of fetal descent into the pelvis in relation to an imaginary line drawn between the ischial spines.

    - Point of maximal impulse (PMI) – The point at which the FHR is heard the loudest.

      - PMI is the optimal location where the fetal heart tones are auscultated the loudest on the woman's abdomen. These tones are best heard directly over the fetal back.

      - In vertex presentation, PMI is either in the right- or left-lower quadrant or below the maternal umbilicus.

      - In breech presentation, PMI is either in the right- or left-upper quadrant above the maternal umbilicus.

- Nursing Actions
  - Preparation of the client
    - Ask the client to empty her bladder before beginning the assessment.
    - Place the client in the supine position with a pillow under her head and have her flex her knees slightly.
    - Place a wedge under her right hip to displace the uterus to the left and prevent supine hypotension/vena cava syndrome.
  - Ongoing care
    - Identify the fetal part occupying the fundus. The head should feel round, firm, and move freely. The breech should feel irregular and soft.
    - Identify the fetal lie and presenting part.
    - Locate and palpate the smooth contour of the fetal back using the palm of one hand and the irregular small parts of the hands, feet, and elbows using the palm of the other hand.
    - Identify the fetal presentation.
    - Determine the fetal presenting part over the true pelvis inlet by gently grasping the lower segment of the uterus between the thumb and fingers. If the head is presenting and not engaged, determine whether the head is flexed or extended.
    - Identify the fetal attitude.
    - Face the client's feet and outline the fetal head using the palmar surface of the fingertips on both hands to palpate the cephalic prominence. If the cephalic prominence is on the same side as the small parts, the head is flexed with vertex presentation. If the cephalic prominence is on the same side as the back, the head is extended with a face presentation.
    - Identify the attitude of the head.
  - Interventions
    - If using an external ultrasound transducer, place the tocotransducer based on the findings obtained from the maneuvers for optimal auscultation of the FHR.
    - Auscultate the FHR postmaneuvers to assess the fetal tolerance to the procedure.
    - Document the findings from the maneuvers.

FHR PATTERN AND UTERINE CONTRACTION MONITORING

- Description of Procedure

  o Intermittent auscultation and uterine contraction palpation

    ▪ Intermittent auscultation of the FHR is a low-technology method that can be performed during labor using a hand-held Doppler ultrasound device, an ultrasound stethoscope, or fetoscope to assess FHR. In conjunction, palpation of contractions at the fundus for frequency, duration, and intensity is used to evaluate fetal well-being. During labor, uterine contractions compress the uteroplacental arteries, temporarily stopping maternal blood flow into the uterus and intervillous spaces of the placenta, decreasing fetal circulation and oxygenation. Circulation to the uterus and placenta resumes during uterine relaxation between contractions. For low-risk labor and delivery, this procedure allows the woman freedom of movement and can be done at home or a birthing center.

    ▪ Follow the facility's policy regarding intermittent auscultation or continuous electronic fetal monitoring.

- Indications

  o Potential diagnoses

    ▪ Rule out labor

    ▪ Active labor

  o Guidelines for intermittent auscultation following routine procedures

    ▪ Rupture of membranes, either spontaneously or artificially

    ▪ Preceding and subsequent to ambulation

    ▪ Prior to and following administration of or a change in medication anesthesia

    ▪ At peak action of anesthesia

    ▪ Following vaginal examination

    ▪ Following expulsion of an enema

    ▪ After urinary catheterization

    ▪ In the event of abnormal or excessive uterine contractions

- Interpretation of Findings

  o A normal, reassuring FHR is 110 to 160/min with increases and decreases from baseline.

- Nursing Actions

  o Preparation of the client

    ▪ Perform Leopold's maneuvers to determine point of maximum impulse (PMI).

    ▪ Auscultate at PMI using listening device.

- Palpate the client's abdomen at uterine fundus to assess uterine activity.
- Count FHR for 30 to 60 seconds to determine baseline rate.
- Auscultate FHR during a contraction and for 30 seconds following the completion of the contraction.

○ Ongoing care

- Identify any nonreassuring FHR patterns and notify the primary care provider.

○ Interventions

- It is the responsibility of the nurse to evaluate FHR patterns, implement nursing interventions, and report nonreassuring patterns to the primary care provider.
- The emotional, educational, and comfort needs of the mother and the family must be incorporated into the plan of care while continuing to assess the FHR pattern's response to the labor process.

○ The method and frequency of fetal surveillance during labor will vary and depend on maternal-fetal risk factors as well as the preference of the facility, primary care provider, and client.

- Description of Procedure

○ Continuous electronic fetal monitoring

- Continuous external fetal monitoring is accomplished by securing an ultrasound transducer over the client's abdomen to determine PMI, which records the FHR pattern, and a tocotransducer on the fundus that records the uterine contractions.
- Advantages of external fetal monitoring
  □ Noninvasive and reduces risk for infection
  □ Membranes do not have to be ruptured
  □ Cervix does not have to be dilated
  □ Placement of transducers can be performed by the nurse
  □ Records permanent record of FHR tracing
- Disadvantages of external fetal monitoring
  □ Contraction intensity is not measurable
  □ Movement of the client requires frequent repositioning of transducers
  □ Quality of recording is affected by client obesity and fetal position

- Indications for Monitoring

○ Potential diagnoses

- Multiple gestations; oxytocin (Pitocin) infusion (augmentation or induction of labor)
- Placenta previa

- Fetal bradycardia
- Maternal complications (diabetes mellitus, preeclampsia, renal disease)
- Intrauterine growth restriction
- Post dates
- Active labor
- Meconium-stained amniotic fluid
- Abruptio placentae – Suspected or actual
- Abnormal nonstress test or contraction stress test
- Abnormal uterine contractions
- Fetal distress

○ Interpretation of findings

- A normal fetal heart rate baseline at term is 110 to 160/min excluding accelerations, decelerations, and periods of marked variability within a 10 min window. At least 2 min of baseline segments in a 10 min window should be present. A single number should be documented instead of a baseline range.
- Fetal heart rate baseline variability is described as fluctuations in the FHR baseline that are irregular in frequency and amplitude. Classification of variability is as follows:
    □ Absent or undetectable variability (considered nonreassuring)
    □ Minimal variability (> undetectable but < 5/min)
    □ Moderate variability (6 to 25/min)
    □ Marked variability (> 25/min)
- Changes in fetal heart rate patterns are categorized as episodic or periodic changes. Episodic changes are not associated with uterine contractions and periodic changes occur with uterine contractions. These changes include accelerations and decelerations.
- According to a report from the 2008 National Institute of Child Health Human Development Workshop, current recommendations for fetal monitoring include a three-tier fetal heart rate interpretation system.
    □ Category I – All of the following are included in the fetal heart rate tracing:
        ‣ Baseline fetal heart rate of 110-160/min
        ‣ Baseline fetal heart rate variability – Moderate
        ‣ Accelerations – Present or absent
        ‣ Early decelerations – Present or absent
        ‣ Variable or late decelerations – Absent

- □ Category II – Category II tracings include all fetal heart rate tracings not categorized as Category I or Category III. Examples of Category II fetal heart rate tracings contain any of the following:
  - ▸ Baseline rate
    - ▷ Tachycardia
    - ▷ Bradycardia not accompanied by absent baseline variability
  - ▸ Baseline FHR variability
    - ▷ Minimal baseline variability
    - ▷ Absent baseline variability not accompanied by recurrent decelerations
    - ▷ Marked baseline variability
  - ▸ Episodic or periodic decelerations
    - ▷ Prolonged fetal heart rate deceleration > 2 min but < 10 min
    - ▷ Recurrent late decelerations with moderate baseline variability
    - ▷ Recurrent variable decelerations with minimal or moderate baseline variability
    - ▷ Variable decelerations with additional characteristics, including "overshoots," "shoulders," or slow return to baseline fetal heart rate
  - ▸ Accelerations
    - ▷ Absence of induced accelerations after fetal stimulation
- □ Category III – Category III fetal heart rate tracings include either:
  - ▸ Sinusoidal pattern
  - ▸ Absent baseline fetal heart rate variability and any of the following:
    - ▷ Recurrent variable decelerations
    - ▷ Recurrent late decelerations
    - ▷ Bradycardia
- ▪ Each uterine contraction is comprised of:
  - □ Increment – The beginning of the contraction as intensity is increasing.
  - □ Acme – The peak intensity of the contraction.
  - □ Decrement – The decline of the contraction intensity as the contraction is ending.
- ▪ Nonreassuring FHR patterns are associated with fetal hypoxia and include:
  - □ Fetal bradycardia.
  - □ Fetal tachycardia.
  - □ Absence of FHR variability.

- Late decelerations.
- Variable decelerations.

FHR PATTERNS	CAUSES/COMPLICATIONS	NURSING INTERVENTIONS
Accelerations (variable transitory increase in the FHR above baseline)	• Healthy fetal/placental exchange • Intact fetal central nervous system (CNS) response to fetal movement • Vaginal exam • Fundal pressure	• Reassuring • No interventions required • Indicate reactive nonstress test
Fetal bradycardia (FHR less than 110/min for 10 min or more)	• Uteroplacental insufficiency • Umbilical cord prolapse • Maternal hypotension • Prolonged umbilical cord compression • Fetal congenital heart block • Anesthetic medications	• Discontinue oxytocin (Pitocin) if it is being infused. • Help the client into a side-lying position. • Administer oxygen (8 to 10 L/min by mask). • Start an IV line if one is not in place. • Administer a tocolytic medication as prescribed. • Stimulate the fetal scalp. • Notify the primary care provider.
Fetal tachycardia (FHR greater than 160/min for 10 min or more)	• Maternal infection, chorioamnionitis • Fetal anemia • Fetal heart failure • Fetal cardiac dysrhythmias • Maternal use of cocaine or methamphetamines • Maternal dehydration	• If maternal fever exists, administer antipyretics as prescribed. • Administer oxygen (8 to 10 L/min by mask). • Give bolus of IV fluids.
Decrease or loss of FHR variability (decrease or loss of irregular fluctuations in the baseline of the FHR)	• Medications that depress the CNS such as narcotics, barbiturates, tranquilizers, or general anesthetics • Fetal hypoxemia with resulting acidosis • Fetal sleep cycle • Congenital abnormalities	• Stimulate the fetal scalp. • Assist primary care provider with application of scalp electrode or fetal blood pH sampling. • Position the client into a left-lateral position.

FHR PATTERNS	CAUSES/COMPLICATIONS	NURSING INTERVENTIONS
Early deceleration of FHR (slowing of FHR with start of contraction with return of FHR to baseline at end of contraction)	• Compression of the fetal head resulting from uterine contraction • Vaginal exam • Fundal pressure	• No intervention required.
Late deceleration of FHR (slowing of FHR after contraction has started with return of FHR to baseline well after contraction has ended)	• Uteroplacental insufficiency causing inadequate fetal oxygenation • Maternal hypotension, abruptio placentae, uterine hyperstimulation with oxytocin (Pitocin)	• Change the client to a side-lying position. • Start an IV line if not in place or increase the IV rate. • Discontinue oxytocin (Pitocin) if being infused. • Administer oxygen 8 to 10 L/min per mask. • Notify the primary care provider. • Prepare for an assisted vaginal birth or cesarean birth.
Variable deceleration of FHR (transitory, abrupt slowing of FHR <110 beats/min, variable in duration, intensity, and timing in relation to uterine contraction)	• Umbilical cord compression • Short cord • Prolapsed cord • Nuchal cord (around fetal neck) • Oligohydramnios	• Change the client's position. • Discontinue oxytocin (Pitocin) if it is being infused. • Administer oxygen at 8 to 10 L/min per mask. • Perform or assist with a vaginal examination. • Assist with an amnioinfusion if ordered.

- Nursing Actions

  - Preparation of the client

    - Use Leopold's maneuvers to locate the fetal presenting part and the optimal location for placement of the ultrasound transducer for the best possible auscultation of FHR.

    - Palpate uterine activity at the fundus to identify proper placement location for the tocotransducer to monitor uterine contractions.

- Ongoing care
  - □ Provide education regarding the procedure to the client and the client's partner during placement and adjustments of the fetal monitor equipment.
  - □ Encourage frequent maternal position changes. Explain to the client that adjustments of the monitor may be necessary with position changes.
  - □ If the client needs to void and can ambulate, and it is not contraindicated, the nurse can disconnect the external monitor for the client to use the bathroom.
  - □ If disconnecting of FHR monitor is contraindicated or internal FHR monitor is being used, the nurse can bring the client a bedpan.

- Description of Procedure
  - ○ Continuous internal fetal monitoring
    - Continuous internal fetal monitoring with a scalp electrode is performed by attaching a small spiral electrode to the presenting part of the fetus to monitor the FHR. The electrode wires are then attached to a leg plate that is placed on the client's thigh and then attached to the fetal monitor.
    - Continuous internal fetal monitoring may be used in conjunction with an intrauterine pressure catheter (IUPC), which is a solid or fluid-filled transducer placed inside the client's uterine cavity to monitor the frequency, duration, and intensity of contractions. The average pressure is usually 50 to 85 mm Hg.
      - □ Advantages of internal fetal monitoring
        - ▸ Early detection of abnormal FHR patterns suggestive of fetal distress
        - ▸ Accurate measurement of uterine contraction intensity
        - ▸ Obesity or maternal and fetal movement does not affect recording
        - ▸ Accurate assessment of FHR variability
        - ▸ Allows greater maternal freedom of movement without compromising tracing
      - □ Disadvantages of internal fetal monitoring
        - ▸ Membranes must have ruptured to use internal monitoring
        - ▸ Cervix must be adequately dilated to a minimum of 2 to 3 cm
        - ▸ Presenting part must have descended enough to place electrode
        - ▸ Potential risk of injury to fetus if electrode is not properly applied
        - ▸ Contraindicated with vaginal bleeding
        - ▸ Potential risk of infection to the client and the fetus
        - ▸ A primary care provider, nurse practitioner/midwife, or specially trained registered nurse must perform this procedure

- Interpretation of Findings

    o A normal, reassuring FHR is 110 to 160/min, with good variability consisting of FHR accelerations above the baseline of at least 15/min, lasting 15 seconds or more with a return to baseline in less than 2 min.

- Nursing Actions

    o Preparation of the client

        ■ Ensure electronic fetal monitoring equipment is functioning properly.

        ■ Continue to monitor FHR patterns.

        ■ Use aseptic techniques if assisting with procedures.

    o Ongoing care

        ■ Monitor maternal vital signs and obtain maternal temperature every 1 to 2 hr.

        ■ Encourage frequent repositioning of the client. If the client is lying supine, place a wedge under one of the client's hips to tilt her uterus.

- Complications

    o Misinterpretation of FHR patterns

    o Maternal or fetal infection if electrode equipment is not correctly applied

    o Fetal trauma if fetal monitoring electrode or IUPC are inserted into the vagina improperly

    o Supine hypotension secondary to maternal position during continuous electronic monitoring

FETAL SCALP BLOOD SAMPLING

- Description of Procedure

    o Fetal scalp blood sampling is performed by obtaining a sample of blood from the fetal scalp through the cervical opening once the cervix has sufficiently dilated and the membranes have ruptured.

        ■ This sampling is obtained to assess the fetal blood gases consisting of the pH, PO_2, and PCO_2.

- Indications

    o Potential diagnoses

        ■ Fetal distress

        ■ High-risk fetus

    o Client presentation

        ■ Nonreassuring FHR (to verify an ominous heart rate pattern on the fetal monitor)

- Nursing Actions

  - Interventions

    - Continue to monitor FHR pattern.

    - Communicate nonreassuring FHR to primary care provider so that a decision can be made whether to perform a fetal scalp blood sampling.

    - Assist with swabbing the fetal scalp with antiseptic prior to the primary care provider performing the scalp puncture.

    - After the procedure, monitor contractions. Monitor for new scalp bleeding.

- Interpretation of Findings

  - The pH will decrease if fetal hypoxia is present. A normal fetal scalp blood pH is 7.25. A finding of < 7.20 is indicative of fetal distress and requires immediate intervention.

FETAL OXYGEN SATURATION MONITORING

- Description of Procedure

  - Fetal oxygen saturation monitoring/fetal pulse oximetry is performed by inserting a specially designed sensor next to the fetal cheek or temple area to assess fetal oxygen saturation ($FSpO_2$).

    - Criteria for use of fetal oxygen saturation

      - Nonreassuring FHR

      - Used in single fetus gestation

      - At least 36 weeks gestation

      - Vertex presentation

      - Ruptured membranes

      - Cervix dilated to at least 2 cm

      - Fetal station at least -2

    - Evaluation of fetal oxygen saturation provides further information to support the decision of whether to allow labor to continue or to intervene with augmentation or preparation of an emergency cesarean birth.

- Indications

  - Potential diagnoses

    - High-risk fetus

    - Fetal distress

  - Client presentation

    - Nonreassuring FHR

- Interpretation of Findings

  ○ Normal FSpO$_2$ is 30 to 70%

- Nursing Actions

  ○ Ongoing care

    ■ Identify potential candidates for fetal oxygen saturation monitoring.

    ■ Assist in interpreting data obtained from fetal oxygen saturation monitoring.

    ■ Assist the primary care provider during the procedure as needed.

    ■ Communicate findings to the primary care provider.

    ■ Document findings and interventions.

(A) APPLICATION EXERCISES

1. A nurse is assisting with the care of a client in active labor. Which of the following will Leopold's maneuvers assist the nurse in determining? (Select all that apply).

   _____ Presenting part

   _____ Fetal attitude

   _____ Fetal lie

   _____ Position of the cervix

   _____ Degree of fetal descent into the pelvis.

2. A nurse is assisting with the care of a client being induced for labor who is being monitored by an external electronic fetal monitor. The nurse notes that the FHR variability is decreased and resembles a straight line. The mother has not had any pain medication. Which of the following should occur first for an internal scalp electrode to be applied? (Select all that apply.)

   _____ Dilation

   _____ Rupture of membranes

   _____ Effacement

   _____ Engagement

   _____ Rotation of the fetus

3. A newly licensed nurse is reviewing a fetal monitor tracing of a client in active labor with the charge nurse. Which of the following should the nurse recognize as being associated with fetal hypoxia? (Select all that apply.)

   _____ Fetal bradycardia

   _____ Fetal tachycardia

   _____ Absence of FHR variability

   _____ Early decelerations

   _____ Variable decelerations

4. A charge nurse is discussing the potential causes of variable decelerations with a newly licensed nurse. Which of the following should she include in the teaching? (Select all that apply.)

   _____ Short umbilical cord

   _____ **Polyhydramnios**

   _____ Umbilical cord compression

   _____ Uteroplacental insufficiency

   _____ Nuchal cord

5. Discuss the advantages and disadvantages of external fetal monitoring.

(A) **APPLICATION EXERCISES ANSWER KEY**

1. A nurse is assisting with the care of a client in active labor. Which of the following will Leopold's maneuvers assist the nurse in determining? (Select all that apply).

__X__	**Presenting part**
__X__	**Fetal attitude**
__X__	**Fetal lie**
_____	Position of the cervix
__X__	**Degree of fetal descent into the pelvis.**

    Using Leopold's maneuvers to palpate the maternal uterus will assist the nurse in determining the presenting part, fetal lie and attitude, and degree of fetal descent into the pelvis. It will also assist in identifying the number of fetuses and expected location of the point of maximal impulse. It does not determine the position of the cervix.

    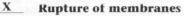

    (N) NCLEX® Connection: Health Promotion and Maintenance, Ante/Intra/Postpartum and Newborn Care

2. A nurse is assisting with the care of a client being induced for labor who is being monitored by an external electronic fetal monitor. The nurse notes that the FHR variability is decreased and resembles a straight line. The mother has not had any pain medication. Which of the following should occur first for an internal scalp electrode to be applied? (Select all that apply.)

__X__	**Dilation**
__X__	**Rupture of membranes**
_____	Effacement
__X__	**Engagement**
_____	Rotation of the fetus

    Prior to the insertion of an internal fetal monitor, the membranes must rupture and the cervix should be dilated approximately 2 to 3 cm. The fetal part should be engaged enough to allow application of the electrode. Effacement and rotation of the fetal presenting part are not necessary prior to application of an internal scalp electrode.

    (N) NCLEX® Connection: Health Promotion and Maintenance, Ante/ Intra/Postpartum and Newborn Care

3. A newly licensed nurse is reviewing a fetal monitor tracing of a client in active labor with the charge nurse. Which of the following should the nurse recognize as being associated with fetal hypoxia? (Select all that apply.)

    __X__   **Fetal bradycardia**

    __X__   **Fetal tachycardia**

    __X__   **Absence of FHR variability**

    _____   Early decelerations

    __X__   **Variable decelerations**

    Fetal bradycardia, fetal tachycardia, variable decelerations, and absence of variability are nonreassuring FHR patterns which are associated with fetal hypoxia. Early decelerations occur with cervical dilation and descent,but are not associated with hypoxia.

 NCLEX® Connection: Health Promotion and Maintenance, Ante/Intra/Postpartum and Newborn Care

4. A charge nurse is discussing the potential causes of variable decelerations with a newly licensed nurse. Which of the following should she include in the teaching? (Select all that apply.)

    __X__   **Short umbilical cord**

    _____   Polyhydramnios

    __X__   **Umbilical cord compression**

    _____   Uteroplacental insufficiency

    __X__   **Nuchal cord**

    A short umbilical cord, umbilical compression, a nuchal cord, and a prolapsed cord may cause variable decelerations. Oligohydramnios, rather than polyhydramnios, causes variable decelerations. Uteroplacental insufficiency results in late decelerations.

 NCLEX® Connection: Health Promotion and Maintenance, Ante/Intra/Postpartum and Newborn Care

5. Discuss the advantages and disadvantages of external fetal monitoring.

    Advantages of external fetal monitoring:

    > **Noninvasive and reduces risk for infection**
    > **Membranes do not have to be ruptured**
    > **Cervix does not have to be dilated**
    > **The nurse can place the transducers**
    > **Records permanent record of FHR tracing**
    > **Disadvantages of external fetal monitoring**
    > **Contraction intensity is not measurable**
    > **Movement of the client requires frequent repositioning of transducers**
    > **Quality of recording is affected by client obesity and fetal position**

 NCLEX® Connection: Health Promotion and Maintenance, Ante/Intra/Postpartum and Newborn Care

UNIT 3: POSTPARTUM NURSING CARE

- Nursing Care of the Client During the Postpartum Period

- Complications of the Postpartum Period

NCLEX® CONNECTIONS
When reviewing the chapters in this section, keep in mind the relevant sections of the NCLEX® outline, in particular:

CLIENT NEEDS: HEALTH PROMOTION AND MAINTENANCE	CLIENT NEEDS: BASIC CARE AND COMFORT	CLIENT NEEDS: REDUCTION OF RISK POTENTIAL

Relevant topics/tasks include:
 	
- Ante/Intra/Postpartum and Newborn Care
  - Perform care of postpartum client.
- Data Collection Techniques
  - Collect baseline physical data.
- Developmental Stages and Transitions
  - Assist client with expected life transition.
	Relevant topics/tasks include:
	
	- Non-Pharmacological Comfort Interventions
	  - Assist in planning comfort interventions for client with impaired comfort.
	- Nutrition and Oral Hydration
	  - Monitor and provide for nutritional needs of client.
		Relevant topics/tasks include:
		
		- Potential for Alterations in Body Systems
		  - Compare current client clinical data to baseline information.
		- Potential for Complications from Surgical Procedures and Health Alterations
		  - Reinforce teaching to prevent complications due to surgery or health alterations.

UNIT 3	POSTPARTUM NURSING CARE
Chapter 11	Nursing Care of the Client During the Postpartum Period

 Overview

- The postpartum period, or puerperium, includes physiological and psychosocial adjustments. This period begins at the start of the fourth stage of labor (1 to 4 hr after the delivery of the placenta) and ends when the body returns to the prepregnant state. This process takes approximately 6 weeks.

- The greatest risks during the postpartum period are hemorrhage, shock, and infection.

- Nurses should perform postpartum data collection per facility protocols. Clients with stable vital signs are usually monitored every 15 min x 4 for the first hour, every 30 min x 2 for the second hr, hourly x 2 for at least 2 hr, then every 4 to 8 hr.

> (M) **View Media Supplement:** Postpartum Data Collection (Video)

- Additional data is collected using the acronym BUBBLE:

  o B – Breasts

  o U – Uterus (fundal height, uterine placement, and consistency)

  o B – Bowel and GI function

  o B – Bladder function

  o L – Lochia (color, odor, consistency, and amount [COCA])

  o E – Episiotomy (edema, ecchymosis, approximation)

- Thermoregulation

  o Data collection

    ▪ Postpartum chill, which occurs in the first 2 hr puerperium, is an uncontrollable shaking chill experienced by clients immediately following birth. Postpartum chill is possibly related to a nervous system response, vasomotor changes, a shift in fluids, and/or the work of labor. This is a normal occurrence unless accompanied by an elevated temperature.

  o Nursing actions

    ▪ Provide clients with warm blankets and fluids.

- o   Client education

    - ■   Assure clients that these chills are a self-limiting common occurrence that will only last a short while.

- •   **Fundus**

    - o   Data collection

        - ■   Physical changes of the uterus include involution of the uterus. Involution occurs with contractions of the uterine smooth muscle, whereby the uterus returns to its prepregnant state. The uterus also rapidly decreases in size from approximately 1,000 g (2.2 lb) to 50 to 60 g (< 2 oz) over a period of 6 weeks with the fundal height steadily descending into the pelvis approximately one fingerbreadth (1 cm) per day.

        - ■   Immediately after delivery, the fundus should be firm, midline with the umbilicus, and approximately at the level of the umbilicus. At 12 hr postpartum, the fundus may be palpated at 1 cm above the umbilicus.

        - ■   Every 24 hr the fundus should descend approximately 1 to 2 cm. It should be halfway between the symphysis pubis and the umbilicus by the sixth postpartum day.

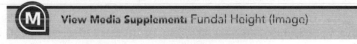
View Media Supplement: Fundal Height (Image)

        - ■   By day 10, the uterus should lie within the true pelvis and should not be palpable.

    - o   Nursing actions

        - ■   Explain the procedure to the client.

        - ■   Apply clean gloves and place a lower perineal pad under the client's buttocks.

        - ■   Cup one hand just above the symphysis pubis to support the lower segment of the uterus, and with the other hand, palpate the client's abdomen to locate the fundus.

            - □   Determine the fundal height by placing fingers on the abdomen and measuring how many fingerbreadths (centimeters) fit between the fundus and the umbilicus above, below, or at the umbilical level.

            - □   Determine if the fundus is midline in the pelvis or displaced laterally (caused by a full bladder).

            - □   Determine if the fundus is firm or boggy. If the fundus is boggy (not firm), lightly massage the fundus in a circular motion.

            - □   Observe lochia flow as the fundus is palpated.

        - ■   Document the fundal height, location, and uterine consistency.

        - ■   Monitor clients receiving oxytocics [oxytocin (Pitocin), methylergonovine maleate (Methergine), and carboprost tromethamine (Hemabate)] to promote uterine contractions and to prevent hemorrhage.

- Monitor for hypotension with oxytocin administration.

- Monitor for hypertension with administration of methylergonovine maleate, ergonovine maleate, and carboprost tromethamine.

  ○ Client education

  - Encourage early breastfeeding for clients who are lactating. This will stimulate the production of natural oxytocin and will help prevent hemorrhage.

  - Encourage frequent emptying of the bladder every 2 to 3 hr to prevent possible uterine displacement and atony.

- Lochia

  ○ Data collection

  - Three stages of lochia (vaginal discharge)

    □ Lochia rubra – Bright red color, bloody consistency, fleshy odor, may contain small clots, transient flow increases during breastfeeding and upon rising. Lasts 1 to 3 days after delivery.

    □ Lochia serosa – Pinkish brown color and serosanguineous consistency. Lasts from approximately day 4 to day 10 after delivery.

    □ Lochia alba – Yellowish, white creamy color, fleshy odor. Lasts from approximately day 11 up to and beyond 6 weeks postpartum.

  - Lochia amount is determined by the quantity of saturation on the perineal pad as being either:

    □ Scant (< 2.5 cm)

    □ Light (< 10 cm)

    □ Moderate (> 10 cm)

    □ Heavy (one pad saturated within 2 hr)

    □ Excessive blood loss (one pad saturated in 15 min or less or pooling of blood under buttocks)

 View Media Supplement: Vaginal Bleeding (Image)

  - Monitor the lochia flow for normal color, amount, and consistency.

    □ Expected findings include

      ▸ Lochia typically trickles from the vaginal opening, but flows more steadily during uterine contractions.

      ▸ A gush of lochia with the expression of clots and dark blood that has pooled in the vagina may occur with ambulation or massage of the uterus.

□ Abnormal findings include

▸ Excessive spurting of bright red blood from the vagina, possibly indicating a cervical or vaginal tear.

▸ Numerous large clots and excessive blood loss (saturation of one pad in 15 min or less), which may be indicative of a hemorrhage.

▸ Foul odor, which is suggestive of an infection.

▸ Persistent lochia rubra in the early postpartum period beyond day three, which may indicate retained placental fragments.

▸ Continued flow of lochia serosa or alba beyond the normal length of time may indicate endometritis, especially if it is accompanied by a fever, pain, or abdominal tenderness.

o Nursing actions

■ Notify the provider.

■ Administer antibiotics if indicated.

■ Assist with emergency care of clients.

o Client education

■ Instruct clients to notify the provider of abnormal findings of lochia.

● Cervix, Vagina, and Perineum

o Data collection

■ The cervix is soft directly after birth and may be edematous, bruised, and have some small lacerations. Within 2 to 3 days postpartum, it shortens and regains its form becoming firm with the os gradually closing.

■ The vagina, which has distended, gradually returns to its prepregnancy size with the reappearance of rugae and a thickening of the vaginal mucosa. However, muscle tone is never restored completely.

■ The soft tissues of the perineum may be erythematous and edematous, especially in areas of an episiotomy or lacerations. Hematomas or hemorrhoids may be present. The pelvic floor muscles may be overstretched and weak.

■ Monitor for cervical, vaginal, and perineal healing.

■ Observe for perineal erythema, edema, and hematoma.

■ Check episiotomy and lacerations for approximation, drainage, quantity, and quality.

□ A bright red trickle of blood from the episiotomy site in the early postpartum period is a normal finding.

o Nursing actions

■ Encourage clients to eat a well-balanced diet, with adequate fruits, vegetables, fiber, and fluids.

- Educate clients about proper cleansing to prevent infection. Tell clients to:
  - Wash hands thoroughly before and after voiding.
  - Use a squeeze bottle filled with warm water or antiseptic solution after each voiding to cleanse the perineal area.
  - Clean the perineal area from front to back (urethra to anus).
  - Blot dry, do not wipe.
  - Use a topical application of antiseptic cream or spray.
  - Change the perineal pad from front to back after voiding or defecating.
- Promote comfort measures.
  - Apply ice packs to the client's perineum for the first 24 to 48 hr to reduce edema and provide anesthetic effect.
  - Encourage sitz baths at a temperature of 38° to 40° C (100° to 104° F) or cooler at least twice a day.
  - Administer analgesia such as nonopioids (acetaminophen [Tylenol]), nonsteroidal anti-inflammatories (ibuprofen [Advil]), and opioids (codeine, hydrocodone) as prescribed for pain and discomfort.
  - Apply topical anesthetics (Americaine spray or Dermoplast) to the client's perineal area as needed or witch hazel compresses (Tuck's) to the rectal area for hemorrhoids.

- Client education
  - Recommend clients to avoid sexual intercourse until the episiotomy/laceration is healed and vaginal discharge has turned white (lochia alba). This usually takes 2 to 4 weeks or until clients are seen by the provider. Over-the-counter lubricants may be needed during the first 6 weeks due to a decrease in estrogen that reduces vaginal lubrication.
  - Inform clients that physiological reactions to sexual activity may be slower and less intense for the first 3 months following birth.
  - Advise clients to begin using contraception upon resumption of sexual activity and that pregnancy can occur while breastfeeding even though menses has not returned.
  - Inform clients who are breastfeeding that menses may not resume for 3 months or until cessation of breastfeeding.
  - Inform clients who are not breastfeeding that menses may not resume until around 4 to 10 weeks.

- Breasts
  - Data collection
    - Secretion of colostrum occurs during pregnancy and 2 to 3 days immediately after birth. Milk is produced 2 to 3 days after the delivery of the newborn.

- ▪ Monitor clients for:
    - □ Redness and tenderness of the breast
    - □ Cracked nipples and indications of mastitis (infection in a milk duct of the breast with concurrent flu-like symptoms)
- ○ Nursing actions
    - ▪ Encourage early-demand breastfeeding, which will also stimulate the production of natural oxytocin and help prevent uterine hemorrhage.
    - ▪ Assist clients into a comfortable position and have her try various positions during breastfeeding (cradle hold, side-lying, and football hold) and explaining how varying positions can prevent nipple soreness.
    - ▪ Reinforce to clients the importance of proper latch techniques (the newborn takes in part of the areola and nipple, not just the tip of the nipple) to prevent nipple soreness.
- ○ Client education
    - ▪ Instruct clients to wear a well-fitting bra continuously for the first 72 hr after birth.
    - ▪ For clients who are lactating
        - □ Emphasize the importance of hand hygiene prior to breastfeeding to prevent infection.
        - □ Instruct clients to:
            - ▸ Completely empty the breasts at each feeding. Massaging the breasts during feeding can help with emptying.
            - ▸ Allow newborns to nurse on demand. Allow newborns to feed 15 to 20 min per breast or until the breast softens. Begin the next breastfeeding session on the breast that was not completely emptied.
        - □ Instruct clients to manage breast engorgement.
        - □ Apply cool compresses between feedings.
        - □ Apply warm compresses or take a warm shower prior to breastfeeding.
        - □ Apply cold cabbage to the breasts to decrease swelling and relieve discomfort.
        - □ Instruct clients with flat nipples to roll the nipples between her fingers just before breastfeeding to help them become more erect and make it easier for newborns to latch on.
        - □ Instruct clients with sore nipples to apply a small amount of breast milk to the nipples and allow it to air-dry after breastfeeding.
        - □ Instruct clients to apply breast creams as prescribed and wear breast shields in their bra to soften the nipples if they are irritated and cracked.
        - □ Encourage clients to consume 2 to 3 L of fluid/day from food and beverage sources to replace fluid lost from breastfeeding, as well as produce an adequate amount of milk for the newborn.

- For nonlactating women

  □ Instruct clients to avoid breast stimulation and running warm water over the breasts for prolonged periods until no longer lactating.

  □ Instruct clients to manage breast engorgement (may occur on the third or fifth postpartum day).

  □ Apply cold compresses 15 min on and 45 min off.

  □ Place fresh cabbage leaves inside the bra.

  □ Take a mild analgesic for pain and discomfort.

- Cardiovascular System and Fluid and Hematologic Status

  o Data collection

  - The cardiovascular system undergoes a decrease in blood volume during the postpartum period related to:

    □ Blood loss during childbirth (average blood loss is 500 mL in an uncomplicated vaginal delivery and 1,000 mL for a cesarean birth).

    □ Diaphoresis and diuresis of the excess fluid accumulated during the last part of the pregnancy. Loss occurs within the first 2 to 3 days postdelivery.

  - Increased Hct and Hgb values are present immediately after delivery for up to 72 hr. Leukocytosis (white blood cell count elevation) of up to 20,000 to 25,000/mm^3 occurs for the first 10 to 14 days without the presence of infection and then returns to normal.

  - Coagulation factors and fibrinogen levels increase during pregnancy and remain elevated for 2 to 3 weeks postpartum. Hypercoagulability predisposes the postpartum woman to thrombus formation and thromboembolism.

  - Blood pressure is usually unchanged with an uncomplicated pregnancy, but may have an insignificant slight transient increase.

  - Possible orthostatic hypotension within the first 48 hr postpartum may occur immediately after standing up with feelings of faintness or dizziness resulting from splanchnic (viscera/internal organs) engorgement that can occur after birth.

  - Elevation of pulse, stroke volume, and cardiac output for the first hour postpartum occurs and then gradually decreases to a prepregnant state baseline by 8 to 10 weeks.

  - Elevation of temperature to 38° C (100° F) resulting from dehydration after labor during the first 24 hr may occur, but should return to normal after 24 hr postpartum.

  o Nursing actions

  - Monitor vital signs per facility protocol.

  - Inspect the client's legs for redness, swelling, and warmth, which are additional signs of venous thrombosis.

  - Encourage early ambulation to prevent venous stasis and thrombosis.

- Apply antiembolism hose to the lower extremities of clients who are at high-risk for developing venous stasis and thrombosis. The hose should be removed as soon as clients are ambulating.

- Administer medications as prescribed.

- Gastrointestinal System and Bowel Function

  - Data collection

    - An increased appetite following delivery

    - Constipation with bowel evacuation delayed until 2 to 3 days after birth

    - Hemorrhoids

  - Nursing actions

    - Monitor clients for reports of hunger.

    - Check for bowel sounds and the return of normal bowel function.

      - Spontaneous bowel movement may not occur for 2 to 3 days after delivery secondary to decreased intestinal muscle tone during labor and puerperium and prelabor diarrhea and dehydration. Clients may also anticipate discomfort with defecation because of perineal tenderness, episiotomy, lacerations, or hemorrhoids.

    - Observe the client's rectal area for varicosities (hemorrhoids).

    - Administer stool softeners (docusate sodium) as prescribed to prevent constipation.

  - Client education

    - Encourage clients to eat a well-balanced diet, with adequate fruits, vegetables, fiber, and fluids.

    - Encourage clients to ambulate.

    - Reinforce the importance of eating a nutritious diet including all food groups. Encourage a diet high in protein, which will aid in tissue repair. Clients should also consume 2 to 3 L of fluid each day from food and beverage sources.

      - Encourage women who are lactating to add an additional daily intake of 330 calories during the first 6 months, and an additional daily intake of 400 calories during the second 6 months.

- Urinary System and Bladder Function

  - Data collection

    - Urinary retention secondary to loss of bladder elasticity and tone and/or loss of bladder sensation resulting from trauma, medications, or anesthesia.

    - A distended bladder as a result of urinary retention can cause uterine atony and displacement to one side, usually to the right. The ability of the uterus to contract is also lessened.

    - Postpartal diuresis with increased urinary output begins within 12 hr of delivery. 1,500 to 3,000 mL/day is expected within the first 2 to 3 days after delivery.

- ○ Nursing actions
  - Determine the client's ability to void every 2 to 3 hr (perineal/urethral edema may cause pain and difficulty in voiding during the first 24 to 48 hr).
  - Observe the client's bladder elimination pattern (client should be voiding every 2 to 3 hr).
  - Monitor clients for signs of a distended bladder
    - □ Fundal height above the umbilicus or baseline level
    - □ Fundus displaced from the midline over to the side
    - □ Bladder bulges above the symphysis pubis
    - □ Excessive lochia
    - □ Tenderness over the bladder area
    - □ Frequent voiding of less than 150 mL of urine is indicative of urinary retention with overflow
  - Insert a straight or indwelling urinary catheter, if necessary, for bladder distention if clients are unable to void to ensure complete emptying of the bladder and allow uterine involution.
- ○ Client education
  - Encourage clients to empty their bladder frequently (every 2 to 3 hr) to prevent possible displacement of the uterus and atony.

- Musculoskeletal System
  - ○ Data collection
    - By 6 to 8 weeks after birth:
      - □ The joints return to their pregnant state and are completely restabilized. The feet however, may remain permanently increased in size.
      - □ Muscle tone begins to be restored throughout the body with the removal of progesterone's effect following delivery of the placenta.
    - The rectus abdominis muscles of the abdomen and the pubococcygeal muscle tone are restored following placental expulsion.
  - ○ Nursing actions
    - Monitor the client's abdominal wall for diastasis recti (a separation of the rectus muscle) anywhere from 2 to 4 cm. It usually resolves within 6 weeks.
  - ○ Client education
    - Reinforce the important of postpartum strengthening exercises, advising them to start with simple exercises, and then gradually progressing to more strenuous ones.
    - Kegel exercises use the same muscles that are used when starting and stopping the flow of urine. Have clients relax and contract the pelvic floor muscles 10 times, eight times a day.

- Pelvic tilt exercises strengthen back muscles and relieve strain on the lower back. Instruct clients to alternately arch and straighten the back.

- Advise clients to use good body mechanics and proper posture.

- Recommend that clients:

  ▸ Not perform housework requiring heavy lifting for at least 3 weeks.

  ▸ Not lift anything heavier than the newborn.

  ▸ Avoid sitting for prolonged periods of time with legs crossed (to prevent thrombophlebitis).

  ▸ Limit stair-climbing for the first few weeks postpartum.

  ▸ Not to drive for the first 2 weeks postpartum, or while taking opioids for pain control.

  ▢ Advise clients who have had a cesarean birth to:

  ▸ Postpone abdominal exercises until about 4 weeks after delivery, or as directed by the provider.

  ▸ Wait until the 6-week follow-up visit before performing strenuous exercise, heavy lifting, or excessive stair-climbing.

- Immune System

  ○ Nursing actions

    - Review rubella status – a client who has a titer of less than 1:8 is administered a subcutaneous injection of rubella vaccine or an measles, mumps and rubella vaccine during the postpartum period to protect a subsequent fetus from malformations. Clients should not get pregnant for 4 weeks following the vaccination.

    - Review hepatitis B status – Newborns born to infected mothers should receive the hepatitis B vaccine and the hepatitis B immune globulin within 12 hr of birth.

    - Review the Rh status – All Rh-negative mothers who have newborns, and are Rh-positive, must be given $RH_o(D)$ immune globulin (RhoGAM) administered IM within 72 hr of the newborn being born to suppress antibody formation in the mother.

  ○ Client education

    - Remind clients who receive both the rubella vaccine and RhoGAM to return to provider after 3 months to determine if immunity to rubella has been developed.

- Comfort and Rest

  ○ Nursing actions

    - Monitor the client's pain level related to episiotomy, lacerations, incisions, afterpains, and sore nipples.

    - Administer pain medications as prescribed.

- ○ Client education

  - ■ Recommend for clients to plan at least one daily rest period and to rest when the newborn sleeps.

- • Maternal Adaptation

  - ○ Data collection

    - ■ Psychosocial adaptation and maternal adjustment begin during pregnancy as clients go through commitment, attachment, and preparation for the birth of the newborn. During the first 2 to 6 weeks after birth, clients go through a period of acquaintance with her newborn, as well as physical restoration. During this time she also focuses on competently caring for her newborn. Finally, the act of achieving maternal identity is accomplished around 4 months following birth. It is important to note that these stages may overlap, and are variable based on maternal, newborn, and environmental factors.

    - ■ Monitor clients for behaviors that facilitate and indicate mother-infant bonding.

      - □ Considers the newborn a family member

      - □ Holds the newborn face to face (en face) maintaining eye contact

      - □ Assigns meaning to the newborn's behavior and views positively

      - □ Identifies the newborn's unique characteristics and relates them to those of other family members

      - □ Touches the newborn and maintains close physical proximity and contact

      - □ Provides physical care for the newborn such as feeding and diapering

      - □ Responds to the newborn's cries

      - □ Smiles at, talks to, and sings to the newborn

    - ■ Monitor clients for behaviors that impair and indicate a lack of mother-infant bonding.

      - □ Apathy when the newborn cries

      - □ Disgust when the newborn voids, stools, or spits up

      - □ Expresses disappointment in the newborn

      - □ Turns away from the newborn

      - □ Does not seek close physical proximity to the newborn

      - □ Does not talk about the newborn's unique features

      - □ Handles the newborn roughly

      - □ Ignores the newborn entirely

    - ■ Monitor clients for signs of mood swings, conflict about maternal role, and/or personal insecurity.

      - □ Feelings of being "down"

      - □ Feelings of inadequacy

- □ Feelings of anxiety related to ineffective breastfeeding

- □ Emotional labiality with frequent crying

- □ Flat affect and being withdrawn

- □ Feeling unable to care for the newborn

- ○ Nursing actions

  - Provide a quiet and private environment that enhances the family bonding process.

  - Facilitate the bonding process by placing the newborn skin-to-skin with the mother soon after birth in an en face position.

  - Encourage the parents to bond with their newborn through cuddling, feeding, diapering, and inspection.

- ○ Client education

  - Provide frequent praise, support, and reassurance to the mother as she moves toward independence in caring for her newborn and adjusting to her maternal role.

  - Encourage the mother/parents to express their feelings, fears, and anxieties about caring for their newborn.

- Paternal Adaptation

  - ○ Data collection

    - Paternal transition to fatherhood consists of a predictable three-stage process during the first few weeks of transition.

      - □ Expectations – The father has preconceived ideas about what it will be like to be a father.

      - □ Reality – The father discovers that his expectations may not be met. Commonly expressed emotions include feeling sad, frustrated, and jealous. He embraces the need to be actively involved in parenting.

      - □ Transition to mastery – The father decides to become actively involved in the care of the newborn.

    - The development of the father-infant bond consists of three stages.

      - □ Making a commitment – The father takes the responsibility of parenting.

      - □ Becoming connected – Experiences feelings of attachment to the newborn.

      - □ Making room for the newborn – The father modifies his life to include the care of the newborn.

- o Nursing actions
  - ▪ Monitor fathers for behaviors that facilitate and indicate father-infant bonding.
    - □ Fathers touch, hold, and maintain eye-to-eye contact with their newborn.
    - □ Fathers observe newborns for features similar to their own to validate claim of the infant.
    - □ Fathers talk and sing to the infant.
  - ▪ Provide education about newborn care when fathers are present.
- o Client education
  - ▪ Assist fathers in their transition to fatherhood by providing guidance and involving him as a full partner rather than just a helper.
  - ▪ Encourage couples to verbalize their concerns and expectations related to newborn care.

- Sibling Adaptation
  - o Data collection
    - ▪ Monitor for positive responses from the sibling.
      - □ Interest and concern for the newborn
      - □ Increased independence
    - ▪ Monitor for adverse responses from the sibling.
      - □ Signs of sibling rivalry and jealousy
      - □ Regression in toileting and sleep habits
      - □ Aggression toward the newborn
      - □ Increased attention-seeking behaviors and whining
  - o Nursing actions
    - ▪ Take siblings on a tour of the obstetric unit.
    - ▪ Encourage the parents to:
      - □ Let siblings be one of the first to see the newborn.
      - □ Provide a gift from the newborn to give the sibling.
      - □ Arrange for one parent to spend time with siblings while the other parent is caring for the newborn.
      - □ Allow older siblings to help in providing care for the newborn.
      - □ Provide toddlers and preschoolers with a doll to care for.

- Family Adaptation

  o Nursing actions

    - Emphasize verbal and nonverbal communication skills between the mother, caregivers, and the infant.

    - Encourage the continued support of grandparents and other family members.

    - Provide information regarding community resources for families with young children.

    - Encourage attendance at parenting classes or support group for new parents. Give the mother/caregivers information about social networks that provide a support system where the mother and caregivers can seek assistance.

- Postpartum Discharge

  o Nursing actions

    - Schedule a postpartum follow-up visit. Following a vaginal delivery, the follow-up visit should take place in 6 weeks, and following a cesarean birth, the visit should take place in 2 weeks.

    - Provide postpartum and newborn instructions in written form.

    - Instruct clients to report danger signs to the provider.

        □ Chills or fever greater than 38° C (100.4° F) for 2 or more days

        □ Change in vaginal discharge with increased amount, large clots, and change to a previous lochia color, such as bright red bleeding and a foul odor

        □ Episiotomy, laceration, or incision pain that does not resolve with analgesics, foul-smelling drainage, redness, and/or edema

        □ Pain or tenderness in the abdominal or pelvic areas that does not resolve with analgesics

        □ Breast(s) with localized areas of pain and tenderness with redness and swelling and/or nipples with cracks or fissures

        □ Calves with localized pain and tenderness, redness, and swelling; a lower extremity with either areas of redness and warmth or coolness and paleness

        □ Urination with burning, pain, frequency, urgency; urine that is cloudy or has blood

        □ Feelings of apathy toward the newborn, inability to provide self- or newborn-care, or feelings that may result in self- or newborn injury

Ⓐ APPLICATION EXERCISES

1. After delivery, the uterus contracts and gradually returns to its prepregnant state. This is referred to as which of the following?

    A. Uterine inversion

    B. Uterine subinvolution

    C. Uterine involution

    D. Uterine exfoliation

2. Explain the three stages of lochia and discuss how to determine the quantity of saturation.

3. A nurse is caring for a client following a spontaneous vaginal birth. The nurse is aware that which of the following hormones decrease after the delivery of the placenta? (Select all that apply.)

    _____ Estrogen

    _____ Progesterone

    _____ Placental enzyme insulinase

    _____ Thyroid stimulating

    _____ Luteinizing hormone

4. A nurse is collecting data from a postpartum client. Which of the following findings indicate signs of bladder distension? (Select all that apply).

    _____ Displaced fundus from midline

    _____ Excessive lochia

    _____ Bladder tenderness

    _____ Fundal height below the umbilicus

    _____ Bulging bladder above the symphysis pubis

5. A nurse is reinforcing interventions to promote comfort to a client with a perineal hematoma. Which of the following statements should the nurse include in the teaching? (Select all that apply.)

    _____ "Apply ice to the perineal area for the first 24 to 48 hr."

    _____ "Use a donut pillow while sitting."

    _____ "Take sitz baths at least twice a day."

    _____ "Use a topical antiseptic cream or spray on the perineal area."

    _____ "Request an indwelling urinary catheter from your provider.

6. A nurse is caring for a family who has a newborn. The father appears to be very anxious and nervous when the newborn's mother asks him to bring her the newborn. Which of the following is an appropriate nursing intervention to promote father infant bonding?

    A. Hand the father the newborn and insist he change the diaper.

    B. Ask the father why he is so anxious and nervous.

    C. Tell the father that he will get used to the newborn in time.

    D. Provide education about newborn care when the father is present.

7. A nurse is caring for a client who is 1 day postpartum. The nurse is collecting data regarding maternal adaptation and mother-infant bonding. Which of the following behaviors indicate the need for nursing intervention?

    A. Demonstrates apathy when the newborn cries.

    B. Identifies and relates newborn's characteristics to family members.

    C. Interprets the newborns behavior as meaningful and a way of expressing needs.

    D. Touches the newborn and maintains close physical proximity.

8. A nurse in the provider's office is caring for a client who is breastfeeding and is 4 days postpartum. The client reports breast engorgement. Which of the following recommendations should the nurse make?

    A. Apply cold cabbage leaves between feedings.

    B. Place warm compresses right after feedings.

    C. Apply breast milk to the nipples and allow them to air dry.

    D. Use the various newborn positions for feedings.

9. A nurse is reinforcing discharge instructions for a client. Which of the following should the nurse instruct the client to report to the provider?

    A. White vaginal discharge

    B. Cramping during breastfeeding

    C. Sore nipple with cracks and fissures

    D. Decreased response with sexual activity

10. A nurse is conducting a home visit with a client who is 3 months postpartum and breastfeeding her newborn. Menses has not yet resumed. The client is discussing contraception with the nurse stating that she does not want to have another child for a couple of years. The nurse understands that this client needs further instruction if the client makes which of the following statements?

    A. "I have already started using the mini-pill for protection."

    B. "Because of our beliefs, we are going to use the rhythm method."

    C. "I am being refitted for a diaphragm with my doctor next week."

    D. "I will not need birth control until I stop breastfeeding."

11. A nurse is reinforcing discharge instructions to a postpartum client following a cesarean birth. The client reports leaking urine every time she sneezes or coughs. Which of the following statements should the nurse include in the teaching?

    A. "Incorporate sit-ups into your exercise routine."

    B. "Begin pelvic tilt exercises to alleviate the leakage."

    C. "Use Kegel exercises to assist with incontinence."

    D. "Try adding abdominal crunches to help with the problem."

APPLICATION EXERCISES ANSWER KEY

1. After delivery, the uterus contracts and gradually returns to its prepregnant state. This is referred to as which of the following?

   A. Uterine inversion

   B. Uterine subinvolution

   C. Uterine involution

   D. Uterine exfoliation

   Uterine involution is the return of the uterus to the prepregnant state. Postpartum contractions aid in uterine involution. Uterine inversion is a condition in which the uterus turns inside out and can be caused by the placenta being removed too vigorously prior to its natural detachment process. Uterine subinvolution is the delay of the uterus in returning to the prepregnancy state. Uterine exfoliation is the shedding of the decidua tissue layers.

   NCLEX® Connection: Physiological Adaptation, Alterations in Body Systems

2. Explain the three stages of lochia and discuss how to determine the quantity of saturation.

   There are three stages of lochia. Lochia rubra is bright red in color with a bloody consistency that may have small clots and lasts 1 to 3 days after birth. Lochia serosa is pinkish brown in color with a serosanguineous consistency and lasts approximately from day four to day 10 after delivery. Lochia alba is yellowish white in color and lasts from approximately day 11 up to and beyond 6 weeks postpartum. The amount of lochia is determined by the quantity of saturation on the perineal pad, with scant being less than 2.5 cm, light less than 10 cm, moderate more than 10 cm, heavy one pad within 2 hr, and excessive one pad within 15 min.

   NCLEX® Connection: Health Promotion and Maintenance, Ante/Intra/Postpartum and Newborn Care

3. A nurse is caring for a client following a spontaneous vaginal birth. The nurse is aware that which of the following hormones decrease after the delivery of the placenta? (Select all that apply.)

X	**Estrogen**
X	**Progesterone**
X	**Placental enzyme insulinase**
_____	Thyroid stimulating
_____	Luteinizing hormone

   After delivery of the placenta, hormones (estrogen, progesterone, and placental enzyme insulinase) decrease, thus resulting in decreased blood glucose, estrogen, and progesterone levels. Thyroid stimulating hormone and luteinizing hormone are not decreased.

   NCLEX® Connection: Physiological Adaptation, Alterations in Body Systems

4. A nurse is collecting data from a postpartum client. Which of the following findings indicate signs of bladder distension? (Select all that apply).

   X   **Displaced fundus from midline**

   X   **Excessive lochia**

   X   **Bladder tenderness**

         Fundal height below the umbilicus

   X   **Bulging bladder above the symphysis pubis**

A distended bladder can cause uterine atony and lateral displacement from the midline, usually to the right. Fundal height above the umbilicus, bulging bladder, excessive lochia rubra, and bladder tenderness are also findings associated with bladder distension. Fundal height below the umbilicus is not a sign of bladder distension.

Ⓝ NCLEX® Connection: Health Promotion and Maintenance, Ante/Intra/Postpartum and Newborn Care

5. A nurse is reinforcing interventions to promote comfort to a client with a perineal hematoma. Which of the following statements should the nurse include in the teaching? (Select all that apply.)

   X   **"Apply ice to the perineal area for the first 24 to 48 hr."**

         "Use a donut pillow while sitting."

   X   **"Take sitz baths at least twice a day."**

   X   **"Use a topical antiseptic cream or spray on the perineal area."**

         "Request an indwelling urinary catheter from your provider.

To promote perineal comfort for a small hematoma, ice should be applied for the first 24 to 48 hr to reduce swelling and provide anesthetic effects. Sitz baths and the use of a topical antiseptic cream or spray should be encouraged. Donuts should be avoided as they result in an increase in pain and discomfort. Use of indwelling urinary catheters is not indicated and can lead to infection.

Ⓝ NCLEX® Connection: Health Promotion and Maintenance, Ante/Intra/Postpartum and Newborn Care

6. A nurse is caring for a family who has a newborn. The father appears to be very anxious and nervous when the newborn's mother asks him to bring her the newborn. Which of the following is an appropriate nursing intervention to promote father-infant bonding?

    A. Hand the father the newborn and insist he change the diaper.

    B. Ask the father why he is so anxious and nervous.

    C. Tell the father that he will get used to the newborn in time.

    D. Provide education about newborn care when the father is present.

    Nursing interventions to assist the father in bonding with the newborn include providing education about newborn care when the father is present. It would not be helpful to push the father into providing care such as changing a diaper without first providing education. Asking the father why he is anxious and nervous, and telling him he will get used to the newborn are both nontherapeutic responses.

    Ⓝ NCLEX® Connection: Health Promotion and Maintenance, Developmental Stages and Transitions

7. A nurse is caring for a client who is 1 day postpartum. The nurse is collecting data regarding maternal adaptation and mother-infant bonding. Which of the following behaviors indicate the need for nursing intervention?

    A. Demonstrates apathy when the newborn cries.

    B. Identifies and relates newborn's characteristics to family members.

    C. Interprets the newborns behavior as meaningful and a way of expressing needs.

    D. Touches the newborn and maintains close physical proximity.

    Demonstrating apathy when the newborn cries is an impaired behavior that shows lack of mother-infant bonding and requires intervention by the nurse. Behaviors that facilitate and indicate mother-infant bonding include viewing the characteristics of the newborn, considering the newborn a family member, identifying the newborn's unique characteristics and relating them to other family members, touching the newborn and maintaining close physical proximity and contact, and assigning a meaning to the newborn's behavior and viewing behaviors positively.

    Ⓝ NCLEX® Connection: Health Promotion and Maintenance, Developmental Stages and Transitions

8. A nurse in the provider's office is caring for a client who is breastfeeding and is 4 days postpartum. The client reports breast engorgement. Which of the following recommendations should the nurse make?

   A. Apply cold cabbage leaves between feedings.

   B. Place warm compresses right after feedings.

   C. Apply breast milk to the nipples and allow them to air dry.

   D. Use the various newborn positions for feedings.

   Cold cabbage leaves applied to the breasts between feedings can help with breast engorgement. Applying warm compresses prior to feedings, not immediately after, can assist with the letdown reflex and milk flow. Breast milk applied to the nipples with air drying and using various positions for feedings help with preventing nipple soreness, but have no effect on breast engorgement.

 NCLEX® Connection: Health Promotion and Maintenance, Ante/Intra/Postpartum and Newborn Care

9. A nurse is reinforcing discharge instructions for a client. Which of the following should the nurse instruct the client to report to the provider?

   A. White vaginal discharge

   B. Cramping during breastfeeding

   C. Sore nipple with cracks and fissures

   D. Decreased response with sexual activity

   A sore nipple that has cracks and fissures is an indication of mastitis. Lochia alba, a white vaginal discharge, is an expected finding from 11 days postpartum to approximately 6 weeks following birth. Oxytocin, which is released with breastfeeding, causes the uterus to contract and may cause discomfort. Physiological reactions to sexual activity may be slower and less intense for the first 3 months following birth.

 NCLEX® Connection: Health Promotion and Maintenance, Ante/Intra/Postpartum and Newborn Care

10. A nurse is conducting a home visit with a client who is 3 months postpartum and breastfeeding her newborn. Menses has not yet resumed. The client is discussing contraception with the nurse stating that she does not want to have another child for a couple of years. The nurse understands that this client needs further instruction if the client makes which of the following statements?

    A. "I have already started using the mini-pill for protection."

    B. "Because of our beliefs, we are going to use the rhythm method."

    C. "I am being refitted for a diaphragm with my doctor next week."

    D. "I will not need birth control until I stop breastfeeding."

Lactating does not prevent pregnancy, even if menses has not yet resumed. Progesterone-only oral contraceptives (mini-pills) are a good form of birth control once lactation has been established. The rhythm method is not as effective, but if the couple chooses this due to their belief system, that is their option. The client is correct in having her diaphragm refitted by her provider, which should be done after a pregnancy and birth or a 7 kg (15 lb) weight change.

  Ⓝ NCLEX® Connection: Health Promotion and Maintenance, Lifestyle Choices

11. A nurse is reinforcing discharge instructions to a postpartum client following a cesarean birth. The client reports leaking urine every time she sneezes or coughs. Which of the following statements should the nurse include in the teaching?

    A. "Incorporate sit-ups into your exercise routine."

    B. "Begin pelvic tilt exercises to alleviate the leakage."

    C. "Use Kegel exercises to assist with incontinence."

    D. "Try adding abdominal crunches to help with the problem."

Kegel exercises consist of the voluntary contraction and relaxation of the pubococcygeal muscle as if to start and stop urine flow. This strengthens the pelvic muscles, which will assist the client in decreasing the stress incontinence that occurs with sneezing and coughing. Sit-ups and crunches are both abdominal exercises that should not be performed until the client's 6-week postpartum follow-up appointment. Pelvic tilt exercises consist of the alternate arching and straightening of the back to strengthen the back muscles and relieve back discomfort.

  Ⓝ NCLEX® Connection: Health Promotion and Maintenance: Ante/Intra/Postpartum and Newborn Care

UNIT 3	POSTPARTUM NURSING CARE
Chapter 12	Complications of the Postpartum Period

Overview

- Postpartum complications are unexpected events or occurrences that may happen during the postpartum period. They include:

    o Superficial and deep vein thrombosis, pulmonary embolus, coagulopathies (idiopathic thrombocytopenic purpura and disseminated intravascular coagulation), postpartum hemorrhage, lacerations and/or hematomas, and postpartum depression. It is imperative for a nurse to have a thorough understanding of each disorder and initiate appropriate nursing interventions to achieve positive outcomes.

DEEP VEIN THROMBOSIS

Overview

- Thrombophlebitis refers to a thrombus that is associated with inflammation.

- Thrombophlebitis of the lower extremities may be of superficial veins or of the deep veins, which are most often of the femoral, saphenous, or popliteal veins.

    o Postpartum clients are at risk for a deep vein thrombosis (DVT) that may lead to a pulmonary embolism.

Data Collection

- Risk Factors

    o Pregnancy

    o Immobility

    o Obesity

    o Smoking

    o Cesarean birth

    o Multiparity

    o Greater than 35 years of age

    o Previous thromboembolism

    o Diabetes mellitus

- Subjective Data
    - Leg pain
    - Chills
- Objective Data
    - Physical assessment findings
        - Unilateral swelling, warmth, and redness
        - Warm extremity
        - Calf tenderness
        - Elevated temperature
        - Cough
        - Tachycardia
- Diagnostic Procedures
    - Noninvasive methods
        - Doppler ultrasound scanning
        - Computed tomography
        - Magnetic resonance imaging

Collaborative Care

- Nursing Care
    - Prevention of thrombophlebitis
        - Initiate early and frequent ambulation during the postpartum period.
        - Instruct clients to avoid prolonged periods of standing, sitting, or immobility.
        - Tell clients to elevate their legs when sitting and to avoid crossing their legs, which will reduce the circulation and exacerbate venous stasis.
        - Recommend for clients to maintain fluid intake of 2 to 3 L of water each day from food and beverage sources to prevent dehydration, which causes circulation to be sluggish.
        - Tell the client to discontinue smoking, which is known to be a risk factor.
        - Measure the client's lower extremities for fitted elastic thromboembolic hose to lower extremities. Provide thigh-high antiembolism stockings for the client at high risk for venous insufficiency.
    - Management of thrombophlebitis
        - Encourage clients to rest.
        - Facilitate bedrest and elevation of the client's extremity above the level of the heart (avoid using a knee gatch or pillow under knees).

- ■ Administer intermittent or continuous warm moist compresses.

- ■ Do NOT massage the affected limb to prevent thrombus from dislodging and becoming an embolus.

- ■ Monitor the client's leg circumferences.

- ■ Administer analgesics (nonsteroidal anti-inflammatory agents).

- ■ Administer anticoagulants for DVT.

- • Medications

    - ○ Heparin

        - ■ Anticoagulant

        - ■ Heparin is given IV to prevent formation of other clots and to prevent enlargement of the existing clot.

    - ○ Nursing considerations

        - ■ Monitor clients receiving heparin by continuous IV infusion.

        - ■ Ensure protamine sulfate is available to counteract excessive anticoagulation.

        - ■ Monitor aPTT.

    - ○ Client education

        - ■ Instruct clients to report bleeding from the gums or nose, increased vaginal bleeding, blood in the urine, and frequent bruising.

    - ○ Warfarin (Coumadin)

        - ■ Anticoagulant

        - ■ Warfarin is used to prevent the formation of blood clots. It is administered orally and is continued by clients for approximately 3 months.

    - ○ Nursing considerations

        - ■ Phytonadione (vitamin K), the warfarin antidote, should be readily available for prolonged clotting times.

        - ■ Monitor pro time (PT) and INR.

    - ○ Client education

        - ■ Instruct clients to watch for bleeding from the gums or nose, increased vaginal bleeding, blood in the urine, and frequent bruising.

- • Care After Discharge

    - ○ Client education

        - ■ Instruct clients to:

            - □ Avoid taking aspirin or ibuprofen (increases bleeding tendencies).

            - □ Use an electric razor for shaving.

            - □ Avoid alcohol use (inhibits warfarin).

- ☐ Brush teeth gently.

- ☐ Avoid rubbing or massaging legs.

- ☐ Avoid periods of prolonged sitting or crossing legs.

- Client Outcomes

  - ○ The client will have restored venous patency.

  - ○ The client will adhere to the medication regimen.

  - ○ The client will not develop pulmonary embolus.

- Complications

  - ○ Pulmonary embolus

    - ■ A pulmonary embolus occurs when fragments or an entire clot dislodges, moves into the circulation and enters the pulmonary artery or one of its branches and lodges in a lung, occluding the vessel and obstructing blood flow.

  - ○ Nursing considerations

    - ■ Monitor clients for chills, apprehension, pleuritic chest pain, dyspnea, and tachypnea.

    - ■ Assist with emergency care of the client.

    - ■ Place clients in a semi-Fowler's position with the head of the bed elevated to facilitate breathing.

    - ■ Administer oxygen to clients by mask.

    - ■ Monitor clients receiving thrombolytic therapy.

COAGULOPATHIES (IDIOPATHIC THROMBOCYTOPENIC PURPURA AND DISSEMINATED INTRAVASCULAR COAGULATION)

Overview

- Idiopathic thrombocytopenic purpura (ITP) is a coagulopathy that is an autoimmune disorder in which the life span of platelets is decreased by antiplatelet antibodies. This can result in severe hemorrhage following a cesarean birth or lacerations.

- Disseminated intravascular coagulation (DIC) is a coagulopathy in which clotting and anticlotting mechanisms occur at the same time.

- Clients are at risk for both internal and external bleeding as well as damage to organs resulting from ischemia caused by microclots.

- Coagulopathies are suspected when the usual measures to stimulate uterine contractions fail to stop vaginal bleeding.

Data Collection

- Risk Factors

  - Risk factors for ITP are genetic factors inherited from parents.

  - Risk factors for DIC that occur secondary to other complications

    - Abruptio placenta

    - Amniotic fluid embolism

    - Missed abortion

    - Fetal death in utero (fetus has died but is retained in the uterus for at least 6 weeks)

    - Severe preeclampsia or eclampsia

    - Septicemia

    - Cardiopulmonary arrest

    - Hemorrhage

    - Hydatidiform mole

- Objective Data

  - Physical assessment findings

    - Unusual spontaneous bleeding from the client's gums and nose (epistaxis)

    - Oozing, trickling, or flow of blood from incision, lacerations, or episiotomy

    - Petechiae and ecchymoses

    - Excessive bleeding from venipuncture, injection sites, or slight traumas

    - Tachycardia, hypotension, and diaphoresis

    - Oliguria

- Laboratory Tests

  - CBC with differential

  - Blood typing and crossmatch

  - Clotting factors

    - Platelet levels (thrombocytopenia)

    - Fibrinogen levels (decreased)

    - PT (increased)

    - Fibrin split product levels (increased)

- Diagnostic Procedures

  - A splenectomy may be performed by the provider if ITP does not respond to medical management.

  - Surgical intervention (hysterectomy) for DIC is performed by the provider as indicated.

Collaborative Care

- Nursing Care

    o Monitor clients for bleeding.

    o Monitor urinary output with indwelling urinary catheter.

    o Provide supplemental oxygen.

    o Prepare clients with ITP for splenectomy.

    o Monitor clients receiving IV fluid replacement and blood and blood products.

    o Monitor laboratory work.

- Client Outcomes

    o The client is injury-free.

UTERINE ATONY

Overview

- Uterine atony results from the inability of the uterine muscle to contract adequately after birth. This can lead to postpartum hemorrhage.

- Risk Factors

    o Retained placental fragments

    o Prolonged labor

    o Oxytocin (Pitocin) induction or augmentation of labor

    o Overdistention of the uterine muscle (multiparity, multiple gestations, polyhydramnios [hydramnios], macrosomic fetus)

    o Precipitate labor

    o Magnesium sulfate administration as a tocolytic

    o Anesthesia and analgesia administration

    o Trauma during labor and birth from operative delivery (forceps-assisted or vacuum-assisted birth, cesarean birth)

Data Collection

- Subjective Data

    o Increased vaginal bleeding

- Objective Data
  - Physical assessment findings
    - A uterus that is larger than normal and boggy with possible lateral displacement on palpation
    - Prolonged lochial discharge
    - Irregular or excessive bleeding
    - Tachycardia and hypotension
    - Skin that is pale, cool, and clammy with poor turgor and pale mucous membranes
  - Diagnostic procedures
    - Bimanual compression or manual exploration of the uterine cavity for retained placental fragments by the primary care provider
    - Surgical management such as a hysterectomy

Collaborative Care

- Nursing Care
  - Ensure that the client's urinary bladder is empty.
  - Monitor:
    - Fundal height, consistency, and location.
    - Lochia for quantity, color, and consistency.
    - Perform fundal massage if indicated.
      - □ If the uterus becomes firm, continue assessing maternal hemodynamic status.
      - □ If uterine atony persists, anticipate surgical intervention, such as a hysterectomy.
  - Express clots that may have accumulated in the uterus, but only after the uterus is firmly contracted.
    - It is critical not to express clots prior to the uterus becoming firmly contracted because pushing on an uncontracted uterus can invert the uterus and result in extensive hemorrhage.
  - Monitor vital signs.
  - Monitor clients receiving IV fluids.

POSTPARTUM HEMORRHAGE

Overview

- Postpartum hemorrhage is considered to occur if clients lose more than 500 mL of blood after a vaginal birth or more than 1,000 mL of blood after a cesarean birth. Two complications that can occur following postpartum hemorrhage include hypovolemic shock and anemia.

Data Collection

- o Risk Factors
  - Uterine atony
  - Complications during pregnancy (e.g., placenta previa, abruptio placentae)
  - Precipitous delivery
  - Administration of magnesium sulfate therapy during labor
  - Lacerations and hematomas
  - Inversion of uterus
  - Subinvolution of the uterus
  - Retained placental fragments
  - Coagulopathies (DIC)
- o Subjective data
  - Increased vaginal bleeding
- o Physical assessment findings
  - Soft, boggy uterus with possible displacement on palpation
  - Blood clots larger than a quarter
  - Perineal pad saturation in 15 min or less
  - Return of lochia rubra once lochia has progressed to serosa or alba
  - Constant oozing, trickling, or frank flow of bright red blood from the vagina
  - Tachycardia and hypotension
  - Skin that is pale, cool, and clammy with poor turgor and pale mucous membranes
  - Oliguria
- o Laboratory tests
  - Hgb and Hct
  - Coagulation profile (PT)
  - Blood type and crossmatch

- o Diagnostic tests
  - ▪ Ultrasound to assess for retained fragments

Collaborative Care

- • Nursing Care
  - o Monitor vital signs.
  - o Identify the source of bleeding.
    - ▪ Monitor fundus for height, firmness, and position. If the uterus is found to be boggy, massage it until it is firm in consistency.
    - ▪ Observe lochia for color, quantity, and clots.
    - ▪ Check for signs of bleeding from lacerations, episiotomy site, or hematomas.
  - o Check bladder for distention.
  - o Measure urinary output with an indwelling urinary catheter.
  - o Monitor clients receiving IV fluid replacement with IV isotonic solutions, such as lactated Ringer's solution or 0.9% sodium chloride, colloid volume expanders, such as albumin and blood products (packed RBCs and fresh frozen plasma).
  - o Provide oxygen to clients at 2 to 3 L/min per nasal cannula to increase RBC saturation.
  - o Monitor oxygen saturation with a pulse oximeter.
  - o Elevate the client's legs to a 20° to 30° angle to increase venous return.
- • Medications
  - o Oxytocin (Pitocin)
    - ▪ Uterine stimulant to promote uterine contractions
  - o Methylergonovine (Methergine)
    - ▪ Classification
      - ▫ Uterine stimulant to promote uterine contractions
  - o Misoprostol (Cytotec)
      - ▫ Uterine stimulant to promote uterine contractions
    - ▪ Therapeutic intent
      - ▫ Controls postpartum hemorrhage.
  - o Carboprost tromethamine (Hemabate)
      - ▫ Uterine stimulant to promote uterine contractions
- • Therapeutic Procedures
  - o Curettage may be necessary if medications fail to cause the release of retained placental fragments.

- Care After Discharge
  - Client education
    - Instruct clients to report excessive vaginal bleeding or a return to a previous color lochia.
    - Instruct clients to limit physical activity to conserve strength.
    - Instruct clients to increase iron and protein intake to promote the rebuilding of RBC volume.
- Client Outcomes
  - The client's vital signs and laboratory results will be within expected reference range limits.
  - The client will not experience complications or injury related to postpartum hemorrhage.

LACERATIONS AND/OR HEMATOMAS

Overview

- Lacerations that occur during labor and birth consist of the tearing of soft tissues in the birth canal and adjacent structures including the cervical, vaginal, vulva, perineal, and/or rectal areas.
- An episiotomy may extend and become a third- or fourth-degree laceration.
- A hematoma is a collection of 250 to 500 mL of clotted blood within tissues that may appear as a bulging bluish mass.
  - Hematomas may occur in the pelvic region or higher up in the vagina or broad ligament.
- Hematomas will present with pain rather than visible bleeding.

Data Collection

- Risk Factors
  - Operative vaginal birth (forceps-assisted, vacuum-assisted birth)
  - Precipitate birth
  - Cephalopelvic disproportion
  - Size (macrosomic infant) and abnormal presentation or position of the fetus
  - Prolonged pressure of the fetal head on the vaginal mucosa
  - Previous scarring of the maternal birth canal from infection, injury, or operation
  - Clients who are nulliparous are at a greater risk for injury due to firmer and less resistant tissue
  - Women who have light skin, especially those with reddish hair, have less distensible tissue than women who are dark skin.

- Subjective Data

  o Feelings of an urge to defecate

  o Difficulty voiding due to pressure on the urethra from a hematoma

  o Physical assessment findings

    ▪ Vaginal bleeding even though the uterus is firm and contracted

    ▪ A continuous slow trickle of bright red blood from the vagina, laceration, or episiotomy

    ▪ Severe perineal or rectal pain or a feeling of pressure in the vagina

  o Diagnostic procedures

    ▪ Repair and suturing of the episiotomy or lacerations; ligation of the bleeding vessel or surgical incision for evacuation of the clotted blood from the hematoma

Collaborative Care

- Nursing Care

  o Monitor vital signs.

  o Inspect the cervix, vagina, perineum, and rectum for lacerations and/or hematomas.

  o Monitor lochia.

  o Apply ice packs to treat small hematomas.

  o Administer pain medication.

  o Encourage sitz baths.

    ▪ Encourage cleansing of the perineal area from front to back with a water bottle filled with warm tap water after voiding and defecation.

- Client Outcomes

  o The client's vital signs and laboratory results will be within expected reference range.

INFECTIONS (ENDOMETRITIS, MASTITIS, AND WOUND INFECTIONS)

Overview

- Postpartum infections are complications that may occur up to 28 days following childbirth, or a spontaneous or induced abortion. Fever of 38° C (100.4° F) or higher for 2 consecutive days during the first 10 days of the postpartum period is indicative of a postpartum infection and requires further investigation. The infection may be present in the bladder, uterus, wound, or breast of a postpartum client. The major complication of puerperal infection is septicemia.

- Uterine infection, mastitis wound infection, and urinary tract infection are examples of postpartum infections. Early identification and prompt treatment are imperative to promote positive outcomes.

ENDOMETRITIS	MASTITIS	WOUND INFECTIONS	URINARY TRACT INFECTIONS (UTI)
• Infection of the uterine lining or endometrium • Usually begins on the second to fifth postpartum day, generally starting as a localized infection at the placental attachment site and spreading to include the entire uterine endometrium	• Infection of the breast involving the interlobular connective tissue and is usually unilateral. Mastitis may progress to an abscess if untreated. • It occurs most commonly in mothers breastfeeding for the first time and well after the establishment of milk flow, which is usually 2 to 4 weeks after delivery. • Staphylococcus aureus is usually the infecting organism.	• Sites of wound infections include cesarean incisions, episiotomies, lacerations, and/or any trauma wounds present in the birth canal following labor and birth. • Often develop after discharge	• A potential complication of a UTI is the progression to pyelonephritis with permanent renal damage leading to acute or chronic renal failure. • E. coli is often the infecting organism.

 View Media Supplement: Mastitis (Image)

Data Collection

- Risk Factors

    - Cesarean birth

    - Retained placental fragments and manual extraction of the placenta

    - Prolonged rupture of membranes, prolonged labor

    - Postpartum hemorrhage

    - Milk stasis from a blocked duct

    - Nipple trauma and cracked or fissured nipples

    - Decrease in breastfeeding frequency due to supplementation with bottle feeding

    - Poor hygiene with inadequate hand hygiene between handling perineal pads and breasts

    - Urinary bladder catheterization

        - Episiotomy, laceration, hematoma

- Subjective Data
  - Puerperal infections
    - Flu-like symptoms such as body aches, chills, fever, and malaise
    - Anorexia and nausea
    - Chills, fever, malaise
  - Endometritis
    - Pelvic pain
  - Mastitis
    - Painful or tender, localized hard mass, and reddened area usually on one breast
  - Wound infection
    - Painful incision
  - Perineal discomfort
    - UTI
    - Reports of urgency, frequency, dysuria, and discomfort in the pelvic area
- Objective Data
  - Physical assessment findings
    - Puerperal infections
      - Elevated temperature of at least 38° C (100° F) for 2 or more consecutive days
      - Tachycardia
    - Endometritis
      - Uterine tenderness and enlargement
      - Dark profuse lochia
      - Lochia that is either malodorous or purulent
    - Mastitis
      - Axillary adenopathy in the affected side (enlarged tender axillary lymph nodes) with an area of inflammation that may be red, swollen, warm, and tender
    - Wound infection
      - Wound warmth, erythema, tenderness, pain, edema, seropurulent drainage, and wound dehiscence (separation of wound or incision edges) or evisceration (protrusion of internal contents through the separated wound edges)
    - UTI
      - Urine (cloudy, blood-tinged, malodorous, sediment)
      - Costovertebral angle tenderness

o   Laboratory tests

- Blood, intracervical, or intrauterine bacterial cultures to reveal the offending organism

- WBC count (leukocytosis)

- RBC sedimentation rate (distinctly increased)

- RBC count (anemia)

- Urinalysis positive for bacteria, blood, protein

Collaborative Care

- Nursing Care

  o   Obtain frequent vital signs and temperature.

  o   Check fundal height, position, and consistency.

  o   Determine the client's pain level.

  o   Observe lochia for color, quantity, and consistency.

  o   Inspect breasts, incisions, episiotomy, and lacerations.

  - Collect vaginal and blood cultures.

  - Monitor administration of IV fluids and antibiotics.

  - Encourage fluid intake of 2 to 3 L/day from food and beverage sources.

  - Administering analgesics as prescribed.

  - Reinforce good hand hygiene techniques.

  - Encourage clients to maintain interaction with infants to facilitate bonding.

  - Provide comfort measures such as warm blankets or warm or cool compresses, sitz baths, perineal care.

  - Perform wound care.

- Medications for endometritis

  o   Clindamycin (Cleocin)

  - It is an antibiotic used in the treatment of bacterial infections

  o   Client education

  - Remind clients to take all the medication as prescribed.

  - Instruct clients to notify the provider of the development of watery, bloody diarrhea.

- Care After Discharge

    o Client education

        - Encourage clients to practice thorough hand hygiene and good maternal perineal hygiene (changing perineal pads from front to back).

        - Encourage clients to consume a diet high in protein to promote tissue-healing.

        - Instruct clients with mastitis to:

            □ Use ice packs or warm packs on her affected breasts for discomfort.

            □ Begin breastfeeding from the unaffected breast first to initiate the letdown reflex in the affected breast that is distended or tender.

            □ Continue breastfeeding frequently (at least every 2 to 4 hr), especially on the affected side. Instruct clients to manually express breast milk or use a breast pump if breastfeeding is too painful. If an abscess forms, it may cause contamination of breast milk. If this occurs, breastfeeding should be stopped and the breasts pumped until resolved.

        - Instruct clients who are breastfeeding to:

            □ Perform hand hygiene prior to breastfeeding.

            □ Change breast pads frequently.

            □ Completely empty each breast during each feeding for prevention of milk stasis. Massaging breast tissue during breastfeeding will encourage the emptying of the breasts.

            □ Allow nipples to air dry.

            □ Wear a well-fitting bra for support.

            □ Reinforce proper infant positioning and latching-on techniques, including both the nipple and the areola. The mother should release the infant's grasp on the nipple prior to removing the infant from the breast.

            □ Encourage clients to get adequate rest and maintain a fluid intake of 2 to 3 L per day.

            □ Instruct clients to report breast tenderness, redness, fever, malaise, urgency, frequency, dysuria, or perineal discomfort not relieved with analgesics.

            □ Instruct clients to complete the entire course of antibiotics.

- Client Outcomes

    o The client will be free of signs of infection as evidenced by vital signs and a WBC that is within normal limits, negative blood cultures.

    o The client's breast will be nontender and without redness.

        - The client's wound will be free of erythema, tenderness, pain, edema, and seropurulent.

POSTPARTUM ADJUSTMENT AND MALADJUSTMENT

Overview

- Postpartum blues can occur in approximately 50 to 70% of women during the first few days after birth and generally continues for up to 10 days. Postpartum blues typically resolves in 10 days without interventions.

- Postpartum depression occurs within 6 months of delivery and is characterized by persistent feelings of sadness and intense mood swings. It occurs in 10 to 15% of new mothers and usually does not resolve without intervention. It is similar to nonpostpartum mood disorders.

- Postpartum psychosis develops within the first 2 to 3 weeks of the postpartum period. Clients who have a history of bipolar disorder are at a higher risk. The symptoms are severe and may include confusion, disorientation, hallucinations, delusions, obsessive behaviors, and paranoia, and client may attempt to harm herself or her infant.

  - A nurse should monitor clients for suicidal or delusional thoughts. The infant should be monitored for failure to thrive secondary to an inability of the mother to provide care for her newborn.

Data Collection

- Risk Factors

  - Hormonal changes with a rapid decline in estrogen and progesterone levels

  - Postpartum physical discomfort and/or pain

  - Individual socioeconomic factors

  - Decreased social support system

  - Anxiety about assuming new role as a mother

  - Unplanned or unwanted pregnancy

  - History of previous depressive episode

  - Low self-esteem

  - History of domestic violence

- Subjective Data

  - Postpartum blues

    - Feelings of sadness

    - Lack of appetite

    - Sleep pattern disturbances

    - Feeling of inadequacies

    - Intense mood swings

    - May experience an intense fear and/or anxiety, anger, and inability to cope with the slightest problems, and become despondent

- o Postpartum depression
  - Feelings of guilt and inadequacies
  - Irritability
  - Anxiety
  - Fatigue persisting beyond a reasonable amount of time
  - Feeling of loss
  - Lack of appetite
  - Persistent feelings of sadness
  - Intense mood swings
  - Sleep pattern disturbances
- o Postpartum psychosis
  - Pronounced sadness
  - Disorientation
  - Confusion
  - Paranoia
- Objective Data
  - o Physical assessment findings
    - Postpartum blues
      - □ Crying
    - Postpartum depression
      - □ Crying
      - □ Weight loss
      - □ Flat affect
    - Postpartum psychosis
      - □ Behaviors indicating hallucinations or delusional thoughts of self-harm or harming the infant

Collaborative Care

- Nursing Care
  - o Monitor interactions between the mother and her newborn. Encourage bonding activities.
  - o Monitor client's mood and affect.
  - o Reinforce with clients that feeling down in the postpartum period is expected and self-limiting. Encourage clients to notify the provider if the condition persists.

- ○ Encourage clients to communicate feelings, validate and address personal conflicts, and reinforce personal power and autonomy.

- ○ Reinforce with clients the importance of adherence with any prescribed antidepressant medication regimen.

- Medications

  - ○ Antidepressants may be prescribed by the provider if indicated based on the client's condition.

- Care After Discharge

  - ○ Nursing actions

    - Schedule a follow-up visit prior to the traditional 6-week postpartum visit for clients who are at risk for developing postpartum depression.

    - Request a referral for a mental health consult if indicated.

    - Provide information about community resources such as La Leche League or support groups for new mothers.

  - ○ Client education

    - Advise clients to get plenty of rest and to nap when the newborn sleeps.

    - Reinforce the importance of the client taking time out for herself.

    - Encourage clients to ask for help from family members.

- Client outcomes

  - ○ The client will report no signs or symptoms of depression.

  - ○ The client will demonstrate healthy interactions with the infant.

ⒶAPPLICATION EXERCISES

1. A nurse is caring for a postpartum client. Which of the following findings are the earliest indications of hypovolemia caused by hemorrhage?

   A. Increasing pulse and decreasing blood pressure

   B. Dizziness and increasing respiratory rate

   C. Cool, clammy skin and pale mucous membranes

   D. Altered mental status and level of consciousness

2. A charge nurse is discussing the risk factors associated with postpartum hemorrhage. Which of the following statements by the nurse indicates a need for additional teaching?

   A. "Precipitous delivery may cause postpartum hemorrhage."

   B. "Lacerations are associated with postpartum hemorrhage."

   C. "Oligohydramnios is associated with postpartum hemorrhage."

   D. "Retained placental fragments may cause a postpartum client to hemorrhage."

3. A nurse is providing care for a postpartum client who is experiencing a postpartum hemorrhage. Which of the following medications may be prescribed by the provider? (Select all that apply.)

   _____ Methylergonovine (Methergine)

   _____ Misoprostol (Cytotec)

   _____ Carboprost tromethamine (Hemabate)

   _____ Hydralazine (Apresoline)

   _____ Oxytocin (Pitocin)

4. A postpartum nurse is caring for a client who has deep vein thrombosis. Which of the following are risk factors for development of this disorder? (Select all that apply.)

   _____ Smoking

   _____ Multiparity

   _____ Diabetes mellitus

   _____ Polyhydramnios

   _____ Maternal age greater than 35

5. A nurse is caring for a client who has DIC. Which of the following postpartum complications should the nurse understand is a risk factor for this client?

   A. Hemorrhage

   B. Thrombophlebitis

   C. Diabetes mellitus

   D. Hyperemesis gravidarum

6. A nurse is providing care for four postpartum clients. Which of the following clients is at the greatest risk for postpartum infection?

    A. A client who experienced a precipitate labor less than 3 hr in duration.

    B. A client with premature rupture of membranes and prolonged labor.

    C. A client who delivered a large-for-gestational-age infant.

    D. A client with a boggy uterus that is not well-contracted and increased bleeding.

7. A client who is breastfeeding has mastitis. Which of the following should the nurse reinforce to the client?

    A. Use a breast pump until condition subsides and stop breastfeeding.

    B. Nurse the infant only on the unaffected breast until resolved.

    C. Completely empty each breast at each feeding.

    D. Wear breast binder until lactation has ceased.

8. A nurse is caring for a client who has urinary tract infection. Which of the following is the typical causative agent of infection?

    A. Staphylococcus aureus

    B. E coli

    C. Klebsiella pneumonia

    D. Clostridium perfringens

9. A nurse is caring for a postpartum client that delivered her third infant 3 days ago. The nurse recognizes that which of the following findings are suggestive of postpartum depression? (Select all that apply.)

    _____ Fatigue

    _____ Insomnia

    _____ Euphoria

    _____ Flat affect

    _____ Crying

(A) APPLICATION EXERCISES ANSWER KEY

1. A nurse is caring for a postpartum client. Which of the following findings are the earliest indications of hypovolemia caused by hemorrhage?

   A. Increasing pulse and decreasing blood pressure

   B. Dizziness and increasing respiratory rate

   C. Cool, clammy skin and pale mucous membranes

   D. Altered mental status and level of consciousness

   A rising pulse rate and decreasing blood pressure are often the first signs of inadequate blood volume. Skin that is cool, clammy, and pale along with pale mucous membranes are changes that occur in the physical status of a client with decreased blood volume, but they are not the first sign of inadequate blood volume. Dizziness and increased respiratory rate are findings that occur in hypovolemia, but they are not the earliest indicator. Altered mental status and changes in level of consciousness are later signs of decreased blood volume which leads to hypoxia and low oxygen saturation.

   (N) NCLEX® Connection: Physiological Adaptation, Alterations in Body Systems

2. A charge nurse is discussing the risk factors associated with postpartum hemorrhage. Which of the following statements by the nurse indicates a need for additional teaching?

   A. "Precipitous delivery may cause postpartum hemorrhage."

   B. "Lacerations are associated with postpartum hemorrhage."

   C. "Oligohydramnios is associated with postpartum hemorrhage."

   D. "Retained placental fragments may cause a postpartum client to hemorrhage."

   Precipitous delivery, lacerations, and retained placental fragments are all associated risk factors for postpartum hemorrhage. Oligohydramnios does not place the client at risk for hemorrhage. Therefore, this response would require additional teaching by the charge nurse.

   (N) NCLEX® Connection: Physiological Adaptation, Alterations in Body Systems

3. A nurse is providing care for a postpartum client who is experiencing a postpartum hemorrhage. Which of the following medications may be prescribed by the provider? (Select all that apply.)

__X__	**Methylergonovine (Methergine)**
__X__	**Misoprostol (Cytotec)**
__X__	**Carboprost tromethamine (Hemabate)**
_____	Hydralazine (Apresoline)
__X__	**Oxytocin (Pitocin)**

   Methylergonovine, misoprostol, carboprost tromethamine, and oxytocin may be prescribed for the management of postpartum hemorrhage. Hydralazine is used in the management of pregnancy-induced hypertension.

   (N) NCLEX® Connection: Pharmacological Therapies, Expected Actions/Outcomes

4. A postpartum nurse is caring for a client who has deep vein thrombosis. Which of the following are risk factors for development of this disorder? (Select all that apply.)

__X__	**Smoking**
__X__	**Multiparity**
__X__	**Diabetes mellitus**
____	Polyhydramnios
__X__	**Maternal age greater than 35**

Risk factors for the development of deep vein thrombosis include pregnancy, immobility, obesity, smoking, cesarean birth, multiparity, previous thromboembolism, diabetes mellitus, and maternal age greater than 35 years. Polyhydramnios is not a risk factor associated with deep vein thrombosis.

(N) NCLEX® Connection: Physiological Adaptation, Alterations in Body Systems

5. A nurse is caring for a client who has DIC. Which of the following postpartum complications should the nurse understand is a risk factor for this client?

A. Hemorrhage

B. Thrombophlebitis

C. Diabetes mellitus

D. Hyperemesis gravidarum

DIC may occur secondary in a client who has a postpartum hemorrhage. Thrombophlebitis, diabetes mellitus, and hyperemesis gravidarum are not risk factors for the development of DIC.

(N) NCLEX® Connection: Physiological Adaptation, Alterations in Body Systems

6. A nurse is providing care for four postpartum clients. Which of the following clients is at the greatest risk for postpartum infection?

A. A client who experienced a precipitate labor less than 3 hr in duration.

B. A client with premature rupture of membranes and prolonged labor.

C. A client who delivered a large-for-gestational-age infant.

D. A client with a boggy uterus that is not well-contracted and increased bleeding.

All of the choices present a risk for postpartum infection. However, premature rupture of membranes with a prolonged labor poses the greatest risk, with an open passage to the uterus for pathogens to enter. Precipitate labor and a large-for-gestational-age infant place the client at risk for trauma and lacerations during delivery. A boggy uterus places the client at risk for hemorrhage and infection. These risks are not as great as the rupture of membranes that exceeds 24 hr prior to delivery, which would be the case in premature rupture of membranes (greater than 24 hr prior to birth) and a prolonged labor.

(N) NCLEX® Connection: Health Promotion and Maintenance, Ante/Intra/Postpartum and Newborn Care

7. A client who is breastfeeding has mastitis. Which of the following should the nurse reinforce to the client?

   A. Use a breast pump until condition subsides and stop breastfeeding.

   B. Nurse the infant only on the unaffected breast until resolved.

   C. Completely empty each breast at each feeding.

   D. Wear breast binder until lactation has ceased.

   Instruct the client to completely empty each breast at each feeding for the prevention of milk stasis, which provides a medium for bacterial growth. Frequent breastfeeding should be encouraged to promote milk flow. The client should be instructed to continue breastfeeding, especially on the affected side. The client should wear a well-fitting bra, not one that is too tight or a binder.

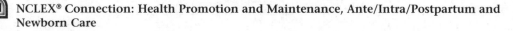 NCLEX® Connection: Health Promotion and Maintenance, Ante/Intra/Postpartum and Newborn Care

8. A nurse is caring for a client who has urinary tract infection. Which of the following is the typical causative agent of infection?

   A. Staphylococcus aureus

   B. E coli

   C. Klebsiella pneumonia

   D. Clostridium perfringens

   E coli is the usual causative agent associated with urinary tract infections. Staphylococcus aureus is usually the infecting organism in mastitis. Klebsiella pneumonia and clostridium perfringens are not associated with urinary tract infections.

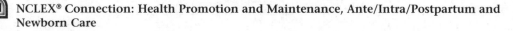 NCLEX® Connection: Health Promotion and Maintenance, Ante/Intra/Postpartum and Newborn Care

9. A nurse is caring for a postpartum client that delivered her third infant 3 days ago. The nurse recognizes that which of the following findings are suggestive of postpartum depression? (Select all that apply.)

X	**Fatigue**
X	**Insomnia**
	Euphoria
X	**Flat affect**
X	**Crying**

   Fatigue, insomnia, flat affect, and bouts of crying spells are findings commonly seen in clients experiencing postpartum depression. Euphoria is not associated with postpartum depression.

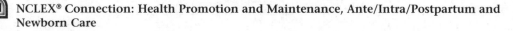 NCLEX® Connection: Health Promotion and Maintenance, Developmental Stages and Transitions

UNIT 4: NEWBORN NURSING CARE

- Newborn Assessment

- Nursing Care of the Newborn

- Complications of the Newborn

NCLEX® CONNECTIONS

When reviewing the chapters in this section, keep in mind the relevant sections of the NCLEX® outline, in particular:

CLIENT NEEDS: HEALTH PROMOTION AND MAINTENANCE

Relevant topics/tasks include:
- Ante/Intra/Postpartum and Newborn Care
  - Contribute to newborn plan of care.
- Data Collection Techniques
  - Prepare client for physical examination.
- Health Promotion/Disease Prevention
  - Identify precautions and contraindications to immunizations.

CLIENT NEEDS: BASIC CARE AND COMFORT

Relevant topics/tasks include:
- Nonpharmacological Comfort Interventions
  - Provide non-pharmacological measures for pain relief.

CLIENT NEEDS: REDUCTION OF RISK POTENTIAL

Relevant topics/tasks include:
- Changes/Abnormalities in Vital signs
  - Check and monitor client vital signs.
- Laboratory Values
  - Monitor diagnostic or laboratory test results.
- Potential for Alterations in Body Systems
  - Identify signs or symptoms of potential prenatal complication.

UNIT 4	NEWBORN NURSING CARE
Chapter 13	Newborn Assessment

Overview

- Apgar scoring, head-to-toe assessment, including vital signs and measurements, gestational age assessment, periods of adjustment to extrauterine life, and diagnostic and therapeutic procedures are components of newborn assessment.

- Newborn assessment occurs at birth (APGAR scoring, quick head-to-toe assessment), upon admission into the nursery, and then before discharge.

- Equipment for Data Collection Following Birth

  o Bulb syringe – Used for the suctioning of excess mucus from the newborn's mouth and nose

  o Stethoscope with a pediatric head – Used to evaluate the newborn's heart rate, breath sounds, and bowel sounds

  o Axillary thermometer – used to monitor the newborn's temperature

  o Blood pressure cuff 2.5 cm wide – For evaluation of the newborn's blood pressure (can use palpation or electronic method)

  o Scale with paper in place – Weight should include pounds and ounces or grams

  o Tape measure with centimeters

  o Clean gloves – Used for examining newborns until the first bath is given

- Initial Data Collection

  o An APGAR score is assigned at 1 and 5 min of life based on 5 assessment parameters.

SCORE	0	1	2
Heart rate	Absent	< 100	> 100
Respiratory rate	Absent	Slow, weak cry	Good cry
Muscle tone	Flaccid	Some flexion	Well-flexed
Reflex irritability	None	Grimace	Cry
Color	Blue, pale	Pink body, cyanotic hands and feet (acrocyanosis)	Completely pink

- 0 to 3 indicates severe distress

- 4 to 6 indicates moderate distress
- 7 to 10 indicates no distress

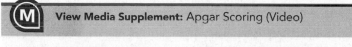

View Media Supplement: Apgar Scoring (Video)

o Head-to-toe exam of newborns within 24 hr of birth

o Obtain vital signs in the following sequence: respirations, heart rate, blood pressure, and temperature.

- Respiratory rate ranges from 30 to 60/min with short periods of apnea (less than 15 seconds). Abnormal findings include periods of apnea lasting longer than 15 seconds, crackles and wheezing (fluid or infection in the lungs), grunting, retractions, and nasal flaring (respiratory distress).

- Heart rate should be 100 to 160/min with brief fluctuations above and below this range depending on activity level (crying, sleeping). Apical pulse rate should be obtained for a full minute, preferably when newborns are sleeping. Place the stethoscope head on the fourth or fifth intercostal space at the left midclavicular line over the apex of the newborn's heart. Report heart murmurs.

- Blood pressure should be 60 to 80 mm Hg systolic and 40 to 50 mm Hg diastolic.

- Temperature should be 36.5° to 37.2° C (97.7 to 98.9° F) axillary. Take an initial rectal per facility policy to check for anal abnormalities. Avoid routine rectal temperatures to prevent injury to rectal mucosa.

o Obtain measurements by measuring the newborn's length from crown to heel of foot for length head circumference at greatest diameter (occipital to frontal). Measure the newborn's chest circumference beginning at the nipple line abdominal circumference above the umbilicus

o Physical exam from head to toe

- Posture

  □ Newborns should be lying in a curled-up position with arms and legs in moderate flexion.

- Skin

  □ Color should be pink or acrocyanotic with no jaundice present on the first day.

  □ Physiological jaundice appears by the third day, but should resolve within a few days.

  □ Good turgor is indicated by skin springing back immediately when pinched.

  □ Texture should be dry, soft, and smooth showing good hydration. Cracks in hands and feet may be present. In full-term newborns, desquamation (peeling) occurs a few days after birth.

  □ Vernix caseosa (protective, thick, cheesy covering) amounts vary, with more present in the newborn's creases and skin folds.

  □ Lanugo (fine downy hair) may be present and is usually found on the newborn's pinnas, forehead, and shoulders.

- □ Normal deviations
  - ▸ Milia (small raised white spots on the nose, chin, and forehead) may be present. These spots disappear spontaneously without treatment (parents should not squeeze the spots).
  - ▸ Mongolian spots (bluish purple spots of pigmentation) are commonly noted on the newborn's shoulders, back, and buttocks. These spots are frequently present on newborns who have dark skin. Be sure the parents are aware of Mongolian spots and notify health care providers of the location and presence of them.
  - ▸ Telangiectatic nevi (stork bites) are flat pink or red marks that easily blanch and are found on the newborn's back of the neck, nose, upper eyelids, and middle of the forehead. They usually fade by the second year of life.
  - ▸ Nevus flammeus (port wine stain) is a capillary angioma below the surface of the skin that is purple or red, varies in size and shape, is commonly seen on the face, and does not blanch or disappear.
  - ▸ Erythema toxicum (erythema neonatorum) is a pink rash that appears suddenly anywhere on the body of a term newborn during the first 3 weeks. This is frequently referred to as newborn rash. No treatment is required.

 View Media Supplement:
  - Mongolian Spots (Image) • Telangiectatic Nevi (Image)

- ■ Head
  - □ Head circumference should be 2 to 3 cm larger than the chest circumference. A head circumference greater than or equal to 4 cm larger than the chest circumference may be an indication of hydrocephalus (excessive cerebral fluid within the brain cavity surrounding the brain). A head circumference less than or equal to 32 cm may be an indication of microcephaly (abnormally small head).
  - □ The anterior fontanel should be approximately 5 cm and diamond shaped. The posterior fontanel is smaller and triangle shaped. Both fontanels should be soft and flat. The fontanels may bulge when the newborn cries, coughs, or vomits and flat when the newborn is quiet. Bulging fontanels may indicate increased intracranial pressure, infection, or hemorrhage. Depressed fontanels may indicate dehydration.
  - □ The sutures of newborns should be palpable, separated, and may be overlapping (molding), a normal occurrence resulting from head compression during labor.

□ Caput succedaneum (localized swelling of the soft tissues of the scalp caused by pressure on the head during labor) is an expected finding that may be palpated as a soft edematous mass and may cross over the suture line. Caput succedaneum usually resolves in 3 to 4 days and does not require treatment.

□ Cephalohematoma is a collection of blood between the periosteum and the skull bone that it covers. It does not cross the suture line. It results from trauma during birth such as pressure of the fetal head against the maternal pelvis in a prolonged difficult labor or forceps delivery. It appears in the first 1 to 2 days after birth and simultaneously resolves in 2 to 3 weeks.

 View Media Supplement:

- Caput Succedaneum (Image) • Cephalohematoma (Image)

- Eyes

  □ Eyes should be symmetrical in size and shape.

  □ Each of the newborn's eyes and the space between them should equal one-third of the total distance between the outer canthus of both eyes to rule out chromosomal abnormalities such as Down syndrome.

  □ Color of eyes is normally blue or gray, with permanent eye color established within 3 to 12 months.

  □ Lacrimal glands are immature in a newborn, resulting in tearless crying.

  □ Subconjunctival hemorrhages may result from pressure during birth.

  □ Pupillary and red reflex should be present.

  □ Eyeball movement will demonstrate random, jerky movements.

- Ears

  □ When examining the placement of the newborn's ears, draw an imaginary line through the inner to the outer canthus of the newborn's eye. The eye should be even with the upper tip of the pinna of the newborn's ear. Ears that are low-set can indicate a chromosome abnormality such as Down syndrome or a renal disorder.

  □ Cartilage should be firm and well-formed. Lack of cartilage indicates prematurity.

  □ Newborns should respond to voices and other sounds.

  □ Inspect the newborn's ears for skin tags.

- Nose

  □ Nose should be midline, flat, and broad with lack of a bridge.

  □ Some mucus should be present, but with no drainage.

  □ Newborn should sneeze to clear his nose.

- Mouth
  - □ The lip movements should be symmetrical with strong suck reflex.
  - □ Saliva should be scant. Excessive saliva may indicate a tracheoesophageal fistula.
  - □ Epstein pearls (small white cysts found on the gums and at the junction of the soft and hard palates) are normal in newborns. They result from the accumulation of epithelial cells and disappear a few weeks after birth.
  - □ The tongue should move freely, be symmetrical in shape, and not protrude (a protruding tongue may be a sign of Down syndrome).
  - □ The soft and hard palate should be intact.
  - □ The gums and tongue should be pink. Gray-white patches on the tongue and gums can indicate thrush, a fungal infection caused by Candida albicans, sometimes acquired from the mother's vaginal secretions.
- Neck
  - □ The neck should be short, thick, surrounded by skin folds, and exhibit no webbing.
  - □ The neck should move freely from side to side and up and down.
  - □ Absence of head control may indicate prematurity or Down syndrome.
- Chest
  - □ The chest should be barrel-shaped.
  - □ Respirations are primarily diaphragmatic without retractions.
  - □ Clavicles should be intact.
  - □ The nipples should be prominent, well-formed, and symmetrical with breast nodules approximately 6 mm. May be edematous related to maternal hormones.
- Abdomen
  - □ The umbilical cord should have two arteries and one vein.
  - □ The umbilical cord should be odorless and exhibit no intestinal structures.
  - □ The abdomen should be round, dome-shaped, and nondistended.
  - □ Bowel sounds should be present 1 to 2 hr following birth.
- Anogenital
  - □ The anus should be present, patent, and not covered by a membrane.
  - □ The genitalia of a male newborn should include rugae on the scrotum, testes descended into the scrotum and the urinary meatus located at penile tip.
  - □ The genitalia of a female should include labia majora covering the labia minora and clitoris. Female genitalia are usually edematous, with a hymenal tag present and possible vaginal blood-tinged discharge, caused by maternal pregnancy hormones.

- □ Urine should be passed within 24 hr after birth. Uric acid crystals will produce a rust color in the urine the first couple of days of life.

- □ Meconium should be passed within 24 hr after birth.

- ■ Extremities

  - □ Full range, symmetry of motion, spontaneous movements and equal length

  - □ Extremities should be flexed with resistance to extension of his extremities.

  - □ No click should be heard when abducting the hips of a newborn.

  - □ Symmetrical gluteal folds, bowed legs and flat feet

  - □ Two-thirds of the soles of the feet should be well-lined.

  - □ The nail beds should be pink without extra digits present.

- ■ Spine

  - □ The newborn's spine should be straight, flat, midline and easily flexed.

  - □ Reflexes

REFLEX	EXPECTED FINDING	EXPECTED AGE
Sucking and rooting reflex	• This reflex is elicited by stroking the newborn's cheek or edge of his mouth. When this is done, the newborn turns his head toward the side that is touched and starts to suck.	Birth to 4 months
Palmar grasp	• This reflex is elicited by placing an object in the newborn's palm. The newborn will grasp the object.	Birth to 6 months
Plantar grasp	• This reflex is elicited by touching the sole of the newborn's foot. The newborn responds by curling his toes downward.	Birth to 8 months
Moro reflex (startle)	• This reflex is elicited by striking a flat surface that the newborn is lying on, or allowing the head and trunk of the newborn in a semisitting position to fall backward to an angle of at least 30°. The newborn's arms and legs symmetrically extend and then abduct while his fingers spread to form a "C."	Birth to 4 months

REFLEX	EXPECTED FINDING	EXPECTED AGE
Tonic neck reflex (fencer position)	• This reflex is elicited by turning a newborn's head to one side. • The newborn will respond by extending his arm and leg on that side, and flex his arm and leg on the opposite side.	Birth to 3 to 4 months
Babinski's reflex	• This reflex is elicited by stroking the outer edge of the newborn's sole of his foot, moving up toward his toes. His toes will fan upward and out.	Birth to 1 year
Stepping	• This reflex is elicited by holding the newborn upright with his feet touching a flat surface. The newborn will respond with stepping movements.	Birth to 4 weeks

 View Media Supplement: Babinski's Reflex (Image)

- Senses
  - Vision – The newborn should be able to focus on objects 9 to 12 in away from his face. This is approximately the distance from the mother's face when the newborn is breastfeeding. The newborn's eyes are sensitive to light; therefore, newborns prefer dim lighting. Pupils are reactive to light and the blink reflex is easily stimulated. The newborn can track high-contrast objects and prefers bright colors and patterns.
  - Hearing – Similar to that of an adult once the amniotic fluid drains from the ears. The newborn turns toward the general direction of a sound.
  - Touch – Newborns should respond to tactile messages of pain and touch.
  - Taste – Newborns can taste and prefer sweets over salty, sour, or bitter.
  - Smell – Newborns have a highly developed sense of smell, prefer sweet smells, and can recognize the smell of their mother.
- Gestational Age Assessment
  - A gestational age assessment is performed within 2 to 12 hr of birth. This assessment involves taking measurements of newborns and the use of the New Ballard Scale. This scale provides an estimation of gestational age and a baseline to assess growth and development.

- ☐ The expected ranges of physical measurements
  - ▸ Weight – 2,500 to 4,000 g (Weigh newborns at the same time daily.)
  - ▸ Length – 45 to 55 cm (18 to 22 inches)
  - ▸ Head circumference – 32 to 36.8 cm (12.6 to 14.5 inches)
  - ▸ Chest circumference – 30 to 33 cm (12 to 13 inches)
- ☐ New Ballard Scale – A newborn maturity rating scale that evaluates neuromuscular and physical maturity. Each individual assessment parameter displays at least six ranges of development along a continuum. Each range of development within an assessment is assigned a number value from -1 to 5. The totals are added to give a maturity rating in weeks gestation (a score of 35 indicates 38 weeks of gestation).
- ☐ Neuromuscular maturity determines:
  - ▸ Posture ranging from fully extended to fully flexed (0 to 4).
  - ▸ Square window formation with the neonate's wrist (-1 to 4).
  - ▸ Arm recoil, where the neonate's arm is passively extended and spontaneously returns to flexion (0 to 4).
  - ▸ Popliteal angle, which is the degree of the angle to which the newborn's knees can extend (-1 to 5).
  - ▸ Scarf sign, which is crossing the neonate's arm over the chest (-1 to 4).
  - ▸ Heel to ear, which is how far the neonate's heels reach to her ears (-1 to 4).
- ☐ Physical maturity determines:
  - ▸ Skin texture, ranging from sticky and transparent, to leathery, cracked, and wrinkled (-1 to 5).
  - ▸ Lanugo presence and amount, ranging from none, sparse, abundant, thinning, bald, or mostly bald (-1 to 4).
  - ▸ Plantar surface creases, ranging from < 40 to 50 mm, to creases over the entire sole (-1 to 4).
  - ▸ Breast tissue amount, ranging from imperceptible to full areola with a 5 to 10 mm bud (-1 to 4).
  - ▸ Eyes and ears for amount of eye opening and ear cartilage present (-1 to 4).
  - ▸ Genitalia development, ranging from flat smooth scrotum to pendulous testes with deep rugae for males (-1 to 4), and prominent clitoris with flat labia to the labia majora covering the labia minora and clitoris for females (-1 to 4).

- Following the physical assessment of newborns, classification of newborns by gestational age and birth weight is then determined.

  - Appropriate for gestational age (AGA) – Weight is between the 10th and 90th percentile

  - Small for gestational age (SGA) – Weight is below the 10th percentile

  - Large for gestational age (LGA) – Weight is above the 90th percentile

  - Low birth weight (LBW) – A weight of 2,500 g or less at birth

  - Intrauterine growth restriction (IUGR) – Growth rate does not meet expected norms

    - Term – Birth between the beginning of week 38 and prior to the end of 42 weeks of gestation

    - Preterm or premature – Born prior to the completion of 37 weeks of gestation

    - Postterm (postdate) – Born after the completion of 42 weeks of gestation

    - Postmature – Born after the completion of 42 weeks of gestation with signs of placental insufficiency

- Periods of Adjustment

  - Observe for periods of reactivity in newborns during the first 6 to 8 hr of life.

    - First period of reactivity – Newborns are alert and exhibit exploring activity, make sucking sounds, and have a rapid heartbeat and respiratory rate. Heart rate may be as high as 160 to 180/min, but will stabilize at a baseline of 100 to 120/min that lasts 15 to 30 min after birth. This is the optimal time for bonding and breastfeeding to take place.

    - Period of relative inactivity – Newborns will become quiet and begin rest and sleep. The newborn's heart rate and respirations will decrease, and this period will last from 30 min to 2 hr after birth.

    - Second period of reactivity – Newborns reawaken, become responsive again, and often gag and choke on mucus that has accumulated in the mouth. This period usually occurs 2 to 8 hr after birth and may last 10 min to several hours.

- Diagnostic and Therapeutic Procedures Following Birth

  - Laboratory tests

    - Hgb and Hct

    - Blood type, Rh-status

    - Glucose for hypoglycemia, per facility policy or order

    - Serum bilirubin

- Phenylketonuria (PKU) testing is required by all states. PKU is a defect in protein metabolism in which the accumulation of the amino acid phenylalanine can result in mental retardation (treatment in the first 2 months of life can prevent retardation). A capillary heel stick should be done 24 hr following birth. For results to be accurate, newborns must receive formula or breast milk for at least 24 hr. If newborns are discharged before 24 hr of age, the test should be repeated in 1 to 2 weeks.

- Other genetic testing that may be done includes: galactosemia, cystic fibrosis, maple syrup urine disease, hypothyroidism, and sickle cell disease.

- Perform heel stick to obtain blood for testing.

  □ Warm the newborn's heel first to increase circulation and eliminate or decrease the pain associated with a heel stick.

  □ Cleanse the newborn's heel with alcohol and allow for drying.

  □ Use a spring-activated lancet so that the skin incision is made quickly and painlessly.

  □ Use the outer aspect of the heel and do not let the lancet go any deeper than 2.4 mm to prevent necrotizing osteochondritis resulting from penetration of bone with the lancet.

  □ Obtain the specimen.

  □ Apply pressure with dry gauze (do not use alcohol as it will cause bleeding to continue) until bleeding stops and cover with an adhesive bandage.

  □ Cuddle and comfort newborns when the procedure is completed to reassure newborns and promote feelings of safety.

EXPECTED LABORATORY VALUES	
Hgb	• 14 to 24 g/dL
Hct	• 44 to 64%
RBC count	• 4,800 to 7,100,000/mm^3
Leukocytes	• 9,000 to 30,000/mm^3
Platelets	• 150,000 to 300,000/mm^3
Glucose	• 40 to 60 mg/dL
Bilirubin	• 0 to 6 mg/dL on day 1 • 8 mg/dL or less on day 2 • 12 mg/dL or less on day 3

- Diagnostic Procedures

  o Newborn hearing screening is required in 46 states, two territories, and the District of Columbia.

Ⓐ **APPLICATION EXERCISES**

1. A nurse is caring for a newborn in the nursery. The newborn weighs 3,200 g and is in the 60th percentile for weight. Apgar scores are 9 and 10 at 1 and 5 min of age. Vital signs are as follows: temperature 37.2° C (99.1° F) axillary, heart rate 160 beats/min, respiratory rate 48/min, length 50.8 cm (20 in), head circumference 35 cm (14 in), and chest circumference 33 cm (13 in). Which of the following is an appropriate classification for the newborn based on weight and gestational age?

   A. LBW

   B. AGA

   C. SGA

   D. LGA

2. A nurse is collecting data from a newborn and observes small white bumps noted on the bridge of the nose. The nurse should document this finding as

   A. Erythema toxicum.

   B. Epstein's pearls.

   C. Mongolian spots.

   D. milia spots.

3. A nurse is assisting a registered nurse with the care of a newborn following a low forceps vaginal delivery. Five minutes after birth, the newborn's heart rate is 110 beats/min. Which of the following Apgar heart rate scores should the newborn receive?

   A. 0

   B. 1

   C. 2

   D. 3

4. A nurse is checking the reflexes of a newborn. Which of the following should the nurse perform to elicit the startle reflex?

   A. Hold the newborn in a semi-sitting position, then allow the newborn's head and trunk to fall backward.

   B. Make a loud noise such as clapping hands together over the newborn's crib.

   C. Stimulate the pads of the newborn's hands with a stroking touch.

   D. Stimulate the soles of the newborn's feet on the outer lateral surface of each foot.

5. A nurse is assisting with the admission of a newborn to the nursery. Which of the following findings indicate that a newborn is experiencing difficulty adapting to extrauterine life? (Select all that apply.)

_____ Grunting

_____ Retractions

_____ Nasal flaring

_____ Apnea for 10 sec periods

_____ Respiratory rate 55/min

6. A nurse is preparing to bathe a newborn and notices a bluish marking across the newborn's lower back. Which of the following is the significance of the finding?

A. The mark is frequently seen in dark-skinned newborns.

B. The mark is abnormal and may indicate hyperbilirubinemia.

C. The mark may be a forceps mark from an operative delivery.

D. The mark is a sign of prolonged birth or trauma during delivery.

APPLICATION EXERCISES ANSWER KEY

1. A nurse is caring for a newborn in the nursery. The newborn weighs 3,200 g and is in the 60th percentile for weight. Apgar scores are 9 and 10 at 1 and 5 min of age. Vital signs are as follows: temperature 37.2° C (99.1° F) axillary, heart rate 160 beats/min, respiratory rate 48/min, length 50.8 cm (20 in), head circumference 35 cm (14 in), and chest circumference 33 cm (13 in). Which of the following is an appropriate classification for the newborn based on weight and gestational age?

    A. LBW

    B. AGA

    C. SGA

    D. LGA

    An AGA newborn's weight is between the 10th and 90th percentile, so this is the proper classification. A LBW newborn would weigh less than 2,500 grams, a SGA newborn's weight is below the 10th percentile, and a LGA newborn's weight is above the 90th percentile.

 NCLEX® Connection: Health Promotion and Maintenance, Data Collection

2. A nurse is collecting data from a newborn and observes small white bumps noted on the bridge of the nose. The nurse should document this finding as

    A. Erythema toxicum.

    B. Epstein's pearls.

    C. Mongolian spots.

    D. milia spots.

    Milia are small white bumps that occur on the nose due to clogged sebaceous glands. Erythema toxicum is a transient maculopapular rash seen in newborns, and Epstein's pearls are small white nodules that appear on the roof a newborn's mouth. Mongolian spots are dark bluish, purple areas noted on the shoulders, back, and buttocks of the newborn. These are frequently observed in dark-skinned newborns.

    NCLEX® Connection: Health Promotion and Maintenance: Ante/Intra/Postpartum and Newborn Care

3. A nurse is assisting a registered nurse with the care of a newborn following a low forceps vaginal delivery. Five minutes after birth, the newborn's heart rate is 110 beats/min. Which of the following Apgar heart rate scores should the newborn receive?

    A. 0

    B. 1

    C. 2

    D. 3

    The 5 min heart rate score should be two since the heart rate is greater than 100.

    NCLEX® Connection: Health Promotion and Maintenance, Data Collection

4. A nurse is checking the reflexes of a newborn. Which of the following should the nurse perform to elicit the startle reflex?

   A. Hold the newborn in a semi-sitting position, then allow the newborn's head and trunk to fall backward.

   B. Make a loud noise such as clapping hands together over the newborn's crib.

   C. Stimulate the pads of the newborn's hands with a stroking touch.

   D. Stimulate the soles of the newborn's feet on the outer lateral surface of each foot.

   Clapping of the hands will elicit the startle reflex in the newborn. Holding the newborn in a semi-sitting position and then allowing the head and trunk to fall backward. Stimulating the pads of the newborn's hands will elicit the grasp reflex. Stimulating the outer lateral portion of the newborn's soles will elicit Babinski's reflex.

   (N) NCLEX® Connection: Health Promotion and Maintenance, Data Collection

5. A nurse is assisting with the admission of a newborn to the nursery. Which of the following findings indicate that a newborn is experiencing difficulty adapting to extrauterine life? (Select all that apply.)

__X__	**Grunting**
X	**Retractions**
X	**Nasal flaring**
_____	Apnea for 10 sec periods
_____	Respiratory rate 55/min

   Grunting, retractions, and nasal flaring are signs of respiratory distress in the newborn. Normal respiratory rate for a newborn increases from 30 to 60/min with short periods of apnea (less than 15 sec). Periods of apnea lasting less than 15 sec are normal.

   (N) NCLEX® Connection: Health Promotion and Maintenance, Data Collection

6. A nurse is preparing to bathe a newborn and notices a bluish marking across the newborn's lower back. Which of the following is the significance of the finding?

   A. The mark is frequently seen in dark-skinned newborns.

   B. The mark is abnormal and may indicate hyperbilirubinemia.

   C. The mark may be a forceps mark from an operative delivery.

   D. The mark is a sign of prolonged birth or trauma during delivery.

   Mongolian spots are commonly found over the lumbosacral area of dark-skinned newborns of African-American, Asian, or Native American origin. Hyperbilirubinemia is present as jaundice. Forceps marks would most likely present as a cephalohematoma, and birth trauma would be present as ecchymosis.

   (N) NCLEX® Connection: Health Promotion and Maintenance: Ante/Intra/Postpartum and Newborn Care

UNIT 4	NEWBORN NURSING CARE
Chapter 14	Nursing Care of the Newborn

Overview

- Nurses play an important role in the care of newborns after birth. Initial nursing care includes maintaining a patent airway, monitoring vital signs, ensuring proper identification, maintaining thermoregulation, monitoring elimination patterns, preventing infection and reinforcing discharge teaching for parents.

- Initial Nursing Care

  o Maintain a patent airway. Keep the bulb syringe with newborns and use it to keep nasal passages clear.

  o Check vital signs at admission/birth and every 30 min x 2, every 1 hr x 2, and then every 8 hr.

  o Monitor newborns for signs and symptoms of respiratory complications.

    ▪ Bradypnea – Respirations less than 25/min

    ▪ Tachypnea – Respirations greater than 60/min

    ▪ Abnormal breath sounds – Expiratory grunting, crackles, and wheezes

    ▪ Respiratory distress – Nasal flaring, retractions, grunting, and labored breathing

  o Obtain daily weights.

    ▪ Ensure proper identification.

  o Identification bands are applied to newborns, usually one on an ankle and one on a wrist, immediately after birth with corresponding bands for mother and significant other, if present. These bands may have permanent locks that must be cut to be removed. Identification bands should include the newborn's name, sex, date, time of birth and mother's hospital number. In addition, the newborn's footprints and mother's thumbprints may be taken. The above information is also included with the footprint sheet.

    ▪ Each time the newborn is taken to his mother, the identification band should be verified against his mother's identification band.

    ▪ All facility staff who assist in caring for newborns are required to wear picture identification badges.

- Newborns are not to be given to anyone who does not have a picture identification badge that distinguishes that person as a staff member of the facility maternal-newborn unit.

- Many facilities have locked maternal-newborn units that require staff to permit entrance or exit. Some facilities have a sensor device on the ID band or umbilical cord clamp that sounds an alarm if the newborn is removed from the facility.

○ Maintain thermoregulation

■ Monitor for signs and symptoms of hypothermia.

□ Axillary temperature less than 36.5° C (97.7° F)

□ Cyanosis

□ Increased respiratory rate

■ Interventions to maintain thermoregulation

□ Maintain temperature between 36.5° C (97.7° F) and 37° C (98.6).

□ To prevent heat loss from conduction, preheat a radiant warmer and warm a stethoscope and other instruments before use, pad a scale with paper before weighing newborns, and place newborns directly on the mother's abdomen and cover with a warm blanket.

▸ To prevent heat loss from convection, place the newborn's bassinet out of the direct line of a fan or air conditioning vent, swaddle newborns in a blanket, and keep the newborn's head covered. Perform procedures under a radiant heat source.

▸ To prevent heat loss of evaporation, rub newborns dry with a warm sterile blanket immediately after delivery, perform the initial bath when the newborn's skin temperature is 36.5° C (97.7° F), perform under a radiant heat source, and expose only one body part at a time, washing and drying thoroughly.

▸ To prevent heat loss from radiation, keep the newborn and examining tables away from windows and air conditioners.

■ Gloves should be worn until the newborn's first bath to avoid exposure to body secretions.

○ Provide nutrition immediately following birth.

■ Initiate breastfeeding as soon as possible after birth to promote maternal-newborn bonding.

■ Start formula feeding at about 2 to 4 hr of age. A few sips of sterile water may be given to check sucking and swallowing reflexes and assure that there are no anomalies such as a tracheoesophageal fistula prior to starting formula feeding.

□ Feed newborns on demand, which is normally every 2 to 3 hr for breastfed newborns and 3 to 4 hr for bottle-fed newborns.

□ Monitor and document feedings per facility protocol.

□ Expect weight loss of 5 to 10% immediately after birth, which should be regained 10 to 14 days after birth.

- Position newborns supine, "back to sleep," to decrease the risk of sudden infant death syndrome.

- Monitor and document elimination patterns.

  □ Newborns should void once within 24 hr of birth. They should void 6 to 10 times a day after 4 days of life.

- Monitor and document the newborn's output.

  □ Meconium should be passed within the first 24 hr after birth. The newborn will then continue to stool 3 to 4 times a day depending on whether he is being breast or bottle-fed.

  □ The stools of newborns who are breastfed may appear yellow and seedy. These stools are lighter in color and looser than the stools of newborns who are formula-fed.

- Keep the perineal area of newborns clean and dry.

  □ Wash the newborn's perineal area after each diaper change with clear water or water with a mild soap. Diaper wipes with alcohol should be avoided. Pat dry and apply triple antibiotic ointment, petroleum jelly, or zinc oxide, depending on facility protocol.

- Prevent infection by providing newborns their own bassinet equipped with a thermometer, diapers, T-shirts, and bathing supplies. Have all personnel caring for a newborn scrub with antimicrobial soap from elbows to finger tips before entering the nursery. Nurses should use proper hand hygiene when caring for newborns. Use cover gowns or special uniforms to avoid direct contact with clothes.

- Monitor umbilical cord. Report a cord that is moist and red, has a foul odor, or has purulent drainage. Remove cord clamp before discharge.

- Family education and promotion of parent-newborn attachment

  □ Provide family education while performing all nursing care. Encourage family involvement, allowing the mother and family to perform newborn care with direct supervision and support by the nurse.

  □ Encourage mothers and family to hold the newborn so that they can experience eye-to-eye contact and interaction.

o Laboratory tests

- Blood glucose levels

- Bilirubin level – Direct and indirect if jaundice is present

- Blood test for genetic screening – All states require testing for phenylketonuria (PKU) and hypothyroidism. Other genetic disorders that may be screened for include galactosemia, cystic fibrosis and maple syrup disease. Blood sample taken at least 24 hr after first feeding.

- o Diagnostic tests

  - Hearing screening – newborns are screened for hearing loss with otoacoustic emissions testing and/or auditory brainstem response. Failure of these screening tests necessitates further testing to make conclusive diagnosis.

- Medications

  - o Erythromycin (Romycin)

    - Prophylactic eye care is the mandatory instillation of antibiotic ointment into the newborn's eyes to prevent ophthalmia neonatorum. Infections can be transmitted during descent through the birth canal. Ophthalmia neonatorum is caused by Neisseria gonorrhoeae or Chlamydia trachomatis and can cause blindness in the newborn.

    - Nursing considerations and client education

      - □ Erythromycin is the medication of choice.

      - □ Apply within 1 to 2 hr of birth.

      - □ Use a single-dose unit to avoid cross-contamination between newborns.

      - □ Apply a 1 to 2 cm ribbon of erythromycin ointment to the lower conjunctival sac of each of the newborn's eyes, starting from the inner canthus and moving outward.

    - Client education

      - □ Reassure the parents that a possible adverse reaction is chemical conjunctivitis, which may cause redness, swelling, drainage, and temporarily blurred vision for 24 to 48 hr and that this will resolve on its own.

  - o Vitamin K (Aquamephyton)

    - This vitamin injection is administered to prevent hemorrhagic disorders. Vitamin K is not produced in the gastrointestinal tract of the newborn until around day 8. Vitamin K is produced in the colon by bacteria that forms once formula or breast milk is introduced into the gut of the newborn.

    - Nursing considerations

      - □ Administer 0.5 to 1 mg IM into the vastus lateralis (where muscle development is adequate) within 1 hr after birth.

  - o Hepatitis B vaccination

    - This immunization provides protection for the newborn against hepatitis B.

    - Nursing considerations

      - □ This immunization is recommended to be given to all newborns.

      - □ For newborns born to healthy women, recommended dosage schedule is at birth, 1 month, and 6 months.

□ For women infected with hepatitis B, hepatitis B immuno globulin (HBIG), along with the hepatitis B vaccine, is given within 12 hr of birth. The hepatitis B vaccine is given alone at 1, 2, and 12 months.

□ Do not give vitamin K and the hepatitis B injections in the same thigh. Sites should be alternated.

- ○ Triple dye
  - ■ Topical antimicrobial may be used for umbilical cord care.
  - ■ Nursing considerations
    - □ Care for the cord as prescribed by the provider. This may include applying triple dye to the umbilical stump or cleansing with sterile water, as recommended by the Association of Women's Health, Obstetrics and Neonatal Nurses. The cord should be kept clean and dry to prevent infection.
  - ■ Therapeutic procedures
    - □ Heel stick blood samples obtained for blood glucose and bilirubin levels and genetic screening
  - ■ Nursing actions
    - □ Warm the newborn's heel to increase circulation.
    - □ Cleanse the newborn's heel with alcohol and allow to dry.
    - □ Use a spring-activated lancet to puncture the skin at the outer aspect of the heel, no deeper than 2.4 mm.
    - □ Collect the blood sample either in a pipet or apply blood to the collection paper.
    - □ Apply pressure with dry gauze (do not use alcohol, as it will cause bleeding to continue) until bleeding stops and cover with an adhesive bandage.
    - □ Cuddle and comfort the newborn when finished.

- • Care of the Newborn at Home
  - ○ Reinforce teaching to parents regarding home care of newborns. Determine previous newborn experience and knowledge, social support available, and educational needs.
  - ○ Crying
    - ■ Inform the parents that newborns cry when they are hungry, overstimulated, wet, cold, hot, tired, bored, or need to be burped. Assure the mother that in time, she will learn what her newborn's cry means. Instruct parents not to feed newborns every time they cry. Overfeeding can lead to stomach aches and diarrhea. It is okay to let a newborn cry for short periods of time.
  - ○ Quieting techniques
    - ■ Swaddling
    - ■ Close skin contact

- Nonnutritive sucking
- Rhythmic noises to simulate utero sounds
- Movement (a car ride, vibrating chair, infant swing, rocking newborn)
- Placing the newborn on his stomach across a holder's lap while bouncing legs
- En face
- Stimulation

○ Sleep-wake cycle

- Instruct parents that most newborns sleep 16 out of every 24 hr the first week at home and sleep 2 to 3 hr at a time. Remind parents to place newborns in the supine position for sleeping.
- Tell parents to keep the newborn's environment quiet and dark at night.
- Discourage parents from allowing newborns in their bed.
- Encourage parents to establish a predictable routine such as bringing newborns out into the center of the action in the afternoon, and keep them there for the rest of the evening. Bathe newborns right before bedtime to provide comfort, give the last feeding around 11 p.m. and then place into a crib or bassinet.
- Suggest that parents keep a small night-light on to avoid having to turn on bright lights when giving nighttime feedings and changing diapers. Encourage parents to speak softly and handle newborns gently so that they go back to sleep easily.

○ Oral and nasal suctioning

- Reinforce to the parents to use a bulb syringe to suction any excess mucus from the newborn's nose and mouth.
- Suction the newborn's mouth first and then the nose, one nostril at a time.
- Compress the bulb syringe before inserting it into the newborn's mouth or nose.
- When suctioning the newborn's mouth, always insert the bulb syringe on the sides of his mouth, not in the middle, and do not touch the back of the throat to avoid eliciting the newborn's gag reflex.

○ Positioning and holding of the newborn

- Reinforce to the parents that newborns have minimal head control. The head must be supported whenever newborns are lifted, especially since the head is larger than the rest of the body.
- Instruct the parents in four basic ways to hold newborns:
  □ Cradle hold – Cradle the newborn's head in the bend of the elbow. This permits eye-to-eye contact (good for feeding).
  □ Upright position – Hold newborns upright and face them toward the holder while supporting the head, upper back, and buttocks (good for burping).

□ Football hold – Support half of the newborn's body in the holder's forearm with the newborn's head and neck resting in the palm of the hand (good for shampooing and breastfeeding).

□ Colic hold – Place newborns face down along the holder's forearm with the hand firmly between the newborn's legs. The newborn's cheek should be by the holder's elbow on the outside. Newborns should be able to see the ground, and the holder's arm should be close to their body, using it to brace and steady newborns (good for quieting a newborn who is fussy).

○ Bathing

■ Instruct the parents to:

□ Cleanse the newborn's face, perineal area, and skin folds daily. Completely bathe the newborn 2 to 3 times a week using mild soap without hexachlorophene.

□ Wash the area around the cord, taking care not to get it wet.

□ Cleanse from the cleanest to dirtiest part of the newborn's body, beginning with his eyes, face, and head; and proceed to the chest, arms, and legs; and wash the groin area last.

□ Do not immerse newborns until the newborn's umbilical cord has fallen off and the circumcision has healed on males.

□ Bathe newborns before a feeding to prevent spitting up or vomiting.

□ Organize all equipment so that newborns are not left unattended in the water (safety). Never leave newborns alone in the tub or sink.

□ Make sure the hot water heater is set at 49° C (120.2° F) or less and that the room is warm. Bath water should be 36.6° to 37.2° C (98° to 99° F). Test the water for comfort on inner wrist prior to bathing newborns.

□ Avoid drafts or chilling of newborns. Expose only the body part being bathed and dry newborns thoroughly.

□ Clean the newborn's eyes using a clean portion of the wash cloth and use clear water to clean each eye. Move from the inner to the outer canthus.

□ Wrap the newborn in a towel and swaddle him in a football hold to shampoo his head.

□ Rinse shampoo from the newborn's head and dry to avoid chilling.

□ In male newborns, to cleanse an uncircumcised penis, wash with soap and water and rinse the penis. The foreskin should not be forced back or constriction may result.

□ In female newborns, wash the vulva by wiping from front to back to prevent contamination of the vagina or urethra from rectal bacteria.

□ Do not use lotions, oils, or powders, because they can alter a newborn's skin and provide a medium for bacterial growth or cause an allergic reaction. Powders may also be inhaled, leading to respiratory issues.

- ○ Feeding
  - ■ Nutritional requirements
    - □ Fluid intake of 100 to 140 mL/kg/24 hr. Newborns should not be given water supplements because they receive enough water from either breast milk or formula.
    - □ For the first 3 months, the newborns require 110 kcal/kg/day. From 3 to 6 months, the requirement decreases to 100 kcal/kg/day. Both breast milk and formula provide 20 kcal/oz. Expect newborns to gain 110 to 200 g/week for the first 3 months.
    - □ Carbohydrates should make up 40% to 50% of the newborn's total caloric intake.
    - □ At least 15% of calories must come from fat (triglycerides). The fat in breast milk is easier to digest than the fat in cow's milk.
    - □ For adequate growth and development to take place, newborns must receive 2.25 to 4 g/kg of protein per day.
    - □ The mineral content of commercial newborn formula and breast milk is adequate with the exception of iron and fluoride.
      - ‣ Iron is low in all forms of milk, but it is absorbed better from breast milk. Newborns who only breastfed for the first 6 months maintain adequate Hgb levels and do not need any additional iron supplementation. After 6 months of age, all newborns need to be fed iron-fortified cereal and other foods rich in iron. Newborns who are formula-fed should receive iron-fortified newborn formula until 12 months of age.
      - ‣ Fluoride levels in breast milk and formulas are low. A fluoride supplement should be given to newborns not receiving fluoridated water after 6 months of age.
    - □ Solids are not introduced until 4 to 6 months of age. If introduced too early, food allergies may develop.
  - ○ Breastfeeding
    - ■ Colostrum is secreted from the mother's breasts during postpartum days 1 to 3. It contains the IgA immunoglobulin that provides passive immunity to the newborns.
    - ■ Breastfeeding is the optimal source of nutrition for newborns. Breastfeeding is recommended exclusively for the first 6 months of age by the American Academy of Pediatrics. Newborns should be breastfed every 2 to 3 hr. Parents should awaken the newborn to feed at least every 3 hr during the day and at least every 4 hr during the night until the newborn is feeding well and gaining weight adequately. Breastfeeding should occur 8 to 12 times within a 24-hr window. Then, a feed-on-demand schedule may be followed.

- Benefits of breastfeeding

    □ Reduces the risk of infection by providing IgA antibodies, lysozymes, leukocytes, macrophages, and lactoferrin that prevent infections.

    □ Promotes rapid brain growth due to large amounts of lactose.

    □ Provides protein and nitrogen for neurological cell building.

    □ Contains electrolytes and minerals.

    □ Breast milk is easy to digest, convenient, and inexpensive.

    □ It improves the newborn's ability to regulate calcium and phosphorus levels.

    □ Sucking associated with breastfeeding reduces dental and ear problems.

- Nursing interventions to promote successful breastfeeding

    □ Explain breastfeeding techniques to mothers, have them perform hand hygiene, get comfortable, and have fluids to drink during breastfeeding.

    □ Offer newborns the breast immediately after birth and frequently thereafter.

    □ Explain the let-down reflex (stimulation of maternal nipple releases oxytocin that causes the letdown of milk).

    □ Reassure mothers that uterine cramps are normal during breastfeeding, resulting from oxytocin.

    □ Instruct mothers to express a few drops of colostrum or milk and spread it over the nipple to lubricate the nipple and entice the newborn.

    □ Show mothers the proper latch-on position. Have them support the breast in one hand with the thumb on top and four fingers underneath. With the newborn's mouth in front of the nipple, the newborn can be stimulated to open his mouth by tickling his lower lip with the tip of the nipple. The mother pulls the newborn to the nipple with his mouth covering part of the areola as well as the nipple.

 View Media Supplement: Breastfeeding Techniques (Images)

    □ Explain to the mother that when her newborn is latched on correctly, his nose, cheeks, and chin will all be touching her breast.

    □ Demonstrate the four basic breastfeeding positions: football, cradle or modified cradle, across the lap, and side-lying.

- Tell mothers to feed newborns 8 to 12 times in a 24-hour period and will usually be on demand or every 2 to 3 hr. Encourage mothers to breastfeed at least 15 to 20 min/breast and 30 to 40 min for the total feeding to ensure that newborns receive adequate fat and protein in rich hind milk. Eventually, newborns will empty a breast within 5 to 10 min, but may need to continue to suck to meet comfort needs.

- Avoid educating mothers regarding the duration of newborn feedings. Clients should be instructed to evaluate when the newborn has completed the feeding, including slowing of newborn suckling, a softened breast, or sleeping.

- Show the mother how to insert a finger in the side of the newborn's mouth to break the suction from the nipple prior to removing the newborn from the breast to prevent nipple trauma.

- Show mothers how to burp newborns when alternating breasts. Newborns should be burped either over the shoulder or in an upright position with the chin supported. Mothers should gently pat newborns on the back to elicit a burp.

- Tell the mother to begin the newborn's next feeding with the breast she stopped feeding with in the previous feeding.

- Tell mothers how to tell if newborns are receiving adequate feeding (gaining weight, voiding 6 to 8 diapers a day, and contentedness between feedings).

- Explain to mothers that newborns may have loose, pale, and/or yellow stools during breastfeeding, and that this is normal.

- Tell mothers how to avoid nipple confusion in newborns by not offering supplemental formula feeding or pacifier. Supplementation can be provided using a small feeding or syringe feeding, if needed.

- If nipples are sore, express breast milk and allow to dry on the breast. The healing properties of the breast milk will decrease soreness and help avoid cracked nipples.

- Tell mothers to always place newborns on the back after feedings.

- Provide instruction for using a breast pump and storing breast milk.

- Recommend the use of a breast pump to provide milk during periods of separation.

    □ Tell mothers that breast pumps can be manual, electric, or battery-operated and pumped directly into a bottle or freezer bag.

    □ Instruct mothers that breast milk may be stored at room temperature for 4 to 6 hr. It may be refrigerated in sterile bottles for use within 8 days, or may be frozen in sterile containers for 3 to 6 months. Breast milk may be stored in a deep freezer for 6 to 12 months.

    □ Tell mothers that thawing the milk in the refrigerator for 24 hr is the best way to preserve the immunoglobulins present in it. It can also be thawed by holding the container under running lukewarm water or placing it in a container of lukewarm water. The bottle should be rotated often, but not shaken when thawing in this manner.

- Tell mothers that thawing by microwave is contraindicated, because it destroys some of the immune factors and lysozymes contained in the milk. Microwave thawing also leads to the development of uneven hot spots in the milk because of uneven heating, which can burn the newborn.

    □ Instruct mothers not to refreeze thawed milk.

    □ Tell mothers to discard used portions of breast milk.

    □ Recommend that mothers avoid consuming alcohol and limit caffeine.

    □ Recommend that mothers only take medications prescribed by the provider.

○ Bottle-feeding

■ Formula feeding can be a successful and adequate source of nutrition if the mother chooses not to breastfeed. The newborn should be fed every 3 to 4 hr. Parents should awaken the newborn to feed at least every 3 hr during the day and at least every 4 hr during the night until the newborn is feeding well and gaining weight adequately. Then, a feed-on-demand schedule may be followed.

■ Nursing interventions to promote successful bottle-feeding

□ Reinforce to parents how to prepare formula, bottles, and nipples.

□ Reinforce to parents about the different forms of formula (ready-to-feed, concentrated, and powder) and how to prepare each correctly.

□ Instruct parents to put bottles in the dishwasher or wash by hand in hot soapy water using a good bottle and nipple brush.

□ Reinforce to parents to wipe the lid clean on the concentrated can before opening it.

□ Instruct parents to use tap water to mix concentrated or powder formula. If the water source is questionable, tap water should be boiled first.

□ Instruct parents that prepared formula can be refrigerated for up to 48 hr.

□ Instruct parents to check the flow of formula from the bottle to assure it is not coming out too slow or too fast.

□ Show parents how to cradle newborns in their arms in a semi-upright position. Newborns should not be placed in the supine position during bottle feeding because of the danger of aspiration. Newborns who bottle-feed do best when held close and at a 45° angle.

□ Instruct parents how to place the nipple on top of the newborn's tongue, to keep the nipple filled with formula to prevent the newborn from swallowing air and to always hold the bottle and never prop it.

□ Instruct parents to burp newborns several times during a feeding, usually after each ½ to 1 oz of formula.

□ Tell parents to place newborns in a supine position after feedings.

□ Tell parents to discard any unused formula remaining in the bottle when newborns are finished feeding due to the possibility of bacterial contamination.

□ Reinforce to parents how to tell if their newborn is being adequately fed (gaining weight, voiding 6 to 8 diapers per day, and satisfaction between feedings).

○ Interventions for newborns at risk for receiving inadequate nutrition

■ Instruct parents who have newborns who are sleepy to:

□ Unwrap newborns.

□ Change the newborn's diaper.

□ Hold newborns upright and turn him from side to side.

- □ Talk to newborns.

- □ Massage the newborn's back, and rub his hands and feet.

- □ Apply a cool cloth to the newborn's face.

- ■ Instruct parents who have newborns who are fussy to:

  - □ Swaddle them.

  - □ Hold them close, move, and rock them gently.

  - □ Reduce the environmental stimuli.

  - □ Place them skin to skin.

- ■ Ensure positioning and latch-on during breastfeeding is correct. Check for maternal allergy to dairy products if breastfed newborn is spitting up, and check for an allergy or intolerance to cow-milk based formula if a bottle-fed newborn is spitting up.

○ Elimination

- ■ Inform parents that newborns should have 6 to 8 wet diapers a day with adequate feedings and may have 3 to 4 stools per day.

- ■ Instruct parents to keep the newborn's diaper area clean and dry. Recommend changing the newborn's diaper frequently, and cleaning the perineal area with warm water or wipes and drying thoroughly to prevent skin breakdown. Apply barrier cream if skin becomes irritated.

○ Cord care

- ■ Instruct parents to:

  - □ Keep the cord dry and keep the top of the diaper folded underneath it.

  - □ Avoid submerging newborns in water until the cord falls off around 10 to 14 days after birth. Give sponge baths until the cord falls off.

  - □ Report any foul smelling, purulent drainage, or redness at the cord site to the provider.

○ Circumcision care

- ■ Circumcision is the surgical removal of the foreskin of the penis.

- ■ Circumcision should not be done immediately following birth because the newborn's level of vitamin K, which prevents hemorrhage, is at a low point and the newborn would be at risk for bleeding.

- ■ Anesthesia is now mandatory for all circumcisions. Types of anesthesia include a ring block, dorsal-penile nerve block, and topical anesthetic (eutectic mixture of local anesthetics). Oral sucrose, oral acetaminophen and nonpharmacologic methods, such as swaddling and nonnutritive sucking, may be employed prior to the procedure. The presence of hypospadias and epispadias are contraindications, because the urethra is located somewhere other than the tip of the urethra, and the foreskin is needed for plastic surgery to repair the defect. Blood disorders, such as hemophilia, are also contraindications due to the increased risk for bleeding.

- The Yellen, Mogen, and Gomco clamp procedures
  - □ The provider applies the Yellen, Mogen, or Gomco clamp to the penis, loosens the foreskin, and inserts the cone under the foreskin to provide a cutting surface for removal of the foreskin and to protect the penis.
  - □ The wound is covered with sterile petroleum gauze to prevent infection and control bleeding.
- The Plastibell procedure
  - □ The provider slides the Plastibell device between the foreskin and the glans of the penis and then ties a suture tightly around the foreskin at the coronal edge of the glans. This applies pressure, as the excess foreskin is removed from the penis.
  - □ After 5 to 7 days, the Plastibell drops off, leaving a clean, well-healed excision.
  - □ No petroleum is used for circumcision with the Plastibell.

 View Media Supplement:
- Circumcision Gomco (Image)   • Circumcision Plastibell (Image)

- Client outcomes
  - □ The newborn will be free of injury following the procedure.
  - □ The newborn will be free from infection following the procedure.
- Preprocedure
  - □ Nursing actions
    - ‣ Collect data to determine any contraindications for the procedure (acute illness, infection, hypospadias or epispadias).
    - ‣ Verify that informed consent has been given.
    - ‣ Keep newborns who are bottle feeding NPO for up to 4 hr prior to the procedure or per facility policy. Breastfed newborns may eat up until the start of the procedure.
- Client education
  - □ Explain the procedure to the parents and assure them that an anesthetic will be administered to minimize pain.
  - □ Explain that the newborn will need to be restrained on a special board during the procedure.

- Intraprocedure
  - □ Nursing actions
    - ▶ Gather and prepare supplies.
    - ▶ Assist with procedure by:
      - ▷ Placing the newborn on the restraining board and restraining the newborn's arms and legs. Do not leave the newborn unattended. Have bulb syringe readily available.
      - ▷ Assisting the provider as needed and comforting the newborn as needed.
      - ▷ Documenting in the nurse's notes circumcision type, date, and time; parent teaching reinforced; any excessive bleeding; and time newborn urinates before discharge.
- Postprocedure care
  - □ Nursing actions
    - ▶ Remove the newborn from the restraining board.
    - ▶ Apply diaper loosely to prevent pressure on the circumcised area.
    - ▶ Check the newborn for bleeding every 15 min for the first hour and then every hour for at least 12 hr.
    - ▶ Ensure the newborn voids.
- Client education
  - □ Reinforce to the parents to keep the area clean. Instruct parents to change the newborn's diaper at least every 4 hr and clean the penis with warm water with each diaper change.
  - □ Instruct parents following clamp procedures to apply petroleum jelly with each diaper change for at least 24 hr after the circumcision to keep the diaper from adhering to the penis.
  - □ Tell parents to apply the diaper loosely to prevent pressure on the circumcised area.
  - □ Instruct parents to not give the newborn a tub bath until the circumcision is completely healed. Until then, warm water should be trickled gently over the penis.
  - □ Tell the parents that a film of yellowish mucus may form over the glans by day 2 and it is important not to wash it off.
  - □ Reinforce to the parents to avoid using premoistened towelettes to clean the penis because they contain alcohol.
  - □ Inform the parents that the newborn may be fussy or may sleep for several hours after the circumcision.
  - □ Inform the parents that the circumcision will heal completely within a couple of weeks.

□ Instruct the parents to notify the provider if there is any redness, discharge, swelling, strong odor, tenderness, decrease in urination, or excessive crying from the newborn.

■ Complications

□ Hemorrhage

■ Nursing actions

□ Monitor the newborn for bleeding.

□ Provide gentle pressure on the penis using 4 x 4 gauze. Gelfoam powder or a sponge may be applied to stop bleeding. If bleeding persists, notify the provider that a blood vessel may need to be ligated. One nurse should continue to hold pressure until the provider arrives while another nurse prepares the circumcision tray and suture material.

□ Provide adequate discharge instructions to the parents about signs and symptoms to observe for and how to report them to the primary care provider.

■ Clothing

□ Instruct the parents about how to properly clothe their newborn. The best clothing is soft and made of cotton. Clothes should be washed separately with mild detergent and hot water. Dress lightly for indoors and on hot days. Too many layers of clothing or blankets can make the newborn too hot. On cold days, cover the newborn's head when outdoors. A general rule is to dress the newborn as the parents would dress themselves.

■ Swaddling

□ Suggest to the parents to swaddle newborns snuggly in a receiving blanket which helps the newborn to feel more secure.

■ Safety

□ Reinforce teaching to parents regarding safety for newborns.

□ Instruct the parents to:

□ Never leave newborns unattended with pets or other small children.

□ Keep small objects (coins) out of the reach of newborns (choking hazard).

□ Never leave newborns alone on a bed, couch, or table. Newborns move enough to reach the edge and fall off.

□ Provide a firm mattress for newborns to sleep on. Never put pillows, large floppy toys, or loose plastic sheeting in a crib. The newborn can suffocate.

□ Not tie anything around the newborn's neck.

□ Monitor the safety of the newborn's crib. The space between the mattress and sides of the crib should be less than 2 fingerbreadths.

□ The slats on the crib should be no more than 2.5 inches apart.

□ Keep the newborn's crib or playpen away from window blinds and drapery cords. Newborns can become strangled in them.

□ Place the bassinet or crib near an inner wall, not next to a window, to prevent cold stress by radiation.

□ Not leave an infant carrier on a high place unattended.

□ Never leave newborns alone during bath time.

□ Have all visitors perform hand hygiene before touching newborns.

□ Keep any individual with an infection away from newborns.

□ Carefully handle newborn. Do not throw newborns up in the air or swing him by his extremities.

□ Encourage parents to:

‣ Have smoke detectors on every floor of a home and to check them monthly to assure that they are working. Batteries should be changed yearly. (Change batteries when daylight savings time occurs or on a child's birthday).

‣ Eliminate potential fire hazards. Keep a crib and playpen away from heaters, radiators, and heat vents. Linens could catch fire if they come into contact with heat sources.

‣ Control the temperature and humidity of the newborn's environment by providing adequate ventilation.

‣ Avoid exposing the newborn to cigarette smoke in a home or elsewhere. Second-hand exposure increases the newborn's risk of developing respiratory illnesses.

■ Car seat safety

□ Instruct the parents to use an approved rear-facing car seat in the back seat, preferably in the middle, (away from air bags and side impact) to transport the newborn. Newborns should be in rear-facing car seats for the first year of life and until they weigh 9.1 kg (20 lb). It is recommended to have the infant ride rear facing until he has reached the weight limit allowed for the car seat as long as the top of his head is below the top of the seat back. In addition, a five-point harness or T-shield should be part of the convertible restraint. Do not use a used or second-hand car seat.

■ Newborn wellness checkups

□ Advise the parents that their newborn will require well-newborn checkups at 2 to 6 weeks of age, and then every 2 months until 6 months of age. Newborns who are breastfed usually have a weight check around 2 days after discharge.

□ Review the schedule for immunizations with the parents.

- Signs of illness to report

  □ Instruct the parents regarding the signs of illness and to report them immediately.

  □ A fever above 38° C (100.4° F) or a temperature below 36.6° C (97.9° F)

  □ Poor feeding or little interest in food

  □ Forceful vomiting or frequent vomiting

  □ Decreased urination

  □ Diarrhea or decreased bowel movements

  □ Labored breathing with flared nostrils or an absence of breathing for greater than 15 seconds

  □ Jaundice

  □ Cyanosis

  □ Lethargy

  □ Inconsolable crying

  □ Difficulty waking

  □ Bleeding or purulent drainage around umbilical cord or circumcision

  □ Drainage developing in eyes.

Ⓐ APPLICATION EXERCISES

1. A nurse is preparing to administer prophylactic eye ointment into the eyes of a newborn to treat ophthalmia neonatorum. Which of the following medications should the nurse anticipate administering?

    A. Ofloxacin (Floxin)

    B. Nystatin (Mycostatin)

    C. Erythromycin (Romycin)

    D. Ceftriaxone (Rocephin)

2. Explain the prescribed treatment for a newborn born to a mother who is infected with hepatitis B.

3. A nurse is providing care to a newborn after birth. Which of the following mechanisms will prevent heat loss from convection? (Select all that apply.)

    _____ Drying the newborn after delivery

    _____ Placing a cap over the newborn's head

    _____ Swaddling the newborn

    _____ Placing the newborn in the radiant warmer

    _____ Placing the newborn's bassinet away from a fan

4. A nurse is providing care for a newborn after birth. Which of the following nursing actions is the highest priority?

    A. Initiating breastfeeding

    B. Determining the newborn's gestational age

    C. Administering a vitamin K injection

    D. Covering the newborn's head with a cap

5. A charge nurse is educating a newly licensed nurse regarding the administration of vitamin K (Aquamephyton) to a newborn. Which of the following is an appropriate response by the nurse to include in the teaching?

    A. "Vitamin K provides immunity."

    B. "Vitamin K assists with blood clotting."

    C. "Vitamin K assists the bowel in maturing."

    D. "Vitamin K prevents cold stress."

6. A nurse is transporting a newborn to his mother following a circumcision. Which of the following security actions should the nurse take?

   A. Validate the newborn's security tag number with the mother's number.

   B. Ask the mother to identify the newborn.

   C. Match the mother's identification band with the newborn's.

   D. Compare the newborn's name on the identification band with the crib card.

7. A nurse is reinforcing teaching to a mother regarding breastfeeding. Which of the following actions by the mother indicates the need for additional teaching?

   A. The mother expresses a few drops of colostrum and places it on her nipple.

   B. The mother inserts a finger in the side of the newborn's mouth before removing the nipple from the newborn's mouth.

   C. The mother gently strokes the newborn's lips with her nipple when she is ready to breastfeed.

   D. The mother places a breast shield over her nipple before placing the nipple in the newborn's mouth.

8. A nurse is reinforcing teaching to a mother about proper techniques for bottle feeding. Which of the following statements made by the mother indicates an understanding of the teaching?

   A. "I will burp my baby at the end of the feeding."

   B. "I should hold my baby close in a supine position."

   C. "I will keep the nipple full of formula throughout the feeding."

   D. "I should refrigerate any unused formula."

9. A nurse is aware that which of the following is a contraindication for circumcising a male newborn? (Select all that apply.)

   _____ Hypospadias

   _____ Hydrocele

   _____ Familiar history of hemophilia

   _____ Hyperbilirubinemia

   _____ Epispadias

10. A nurse is reinforcing discharge teaching to the parents of a newborn. Which of the following statements made by the parents requires additional education?

    A. "I should keep my baby's cord dry and clean with the diaper folded below it."

    B. "I will not remove the yellow exudate that will form on my baby's circumcision."

    C. "I will place my baby's car seat in the back seat in a semi-reclined, rear-facing position."

    D. "I should give my baby some water until my breast milk comes in."

11. A nurse is educating a mother about the proper use of the bulb syringe. Which of the following responses should the nurse include in the teaching?

     A. "Suction the baby's mouth before her nose."

     B. "Suction the baby's nose before her mouth."

     C. "Place the bulb syringe to the back of the baby's throat."

     D. "Compress the syringe after it is placed in the baby's mouth or nose."

(A) **APPLICATION EXERCISES ANSWER KEY**

1. A nurse is preparing to administer prophylactic eye ointment into the eyes of a newborn to treat ophthalmia neonatorum. Which of the following medications should the nurse anticipate administering?

   A. Ofloxacin (Floxin)

   B. Nystatin (Mycostatin)

   C. Erythromycin (Romycin)

   D. Ceftriaxone (Rocephin)

   The medication of choice for ophthalmia neonatorum is erythromycin ophthalmic ointment 0.5%. This antibiotic provides prophylaxis against *Neisseria gonorrhoeae* and *Chlamydia trachomatis*. Ofloxacin is an antibiotic also, but is not used for ophthalmia neonatorum. Nystatin is used for **Candida albicans** in oral yeast infections. Ceftriaxone is an antibiotic, but it is not used for ophthalmia neonatorum.

(N) **NCLEX® Connection: Pharmacological Therapies, Expected Actions/Outcomes**

2. Explain the prescribed treatment for a newborn born to a mother who is infected with hepatitis B.

   If a newborn is born to a mother who is infected with hepatitis B, the newborn should receive the hepatitis B and the hepatitis B immuno globulin (HBIG) vaccines. Both should be administered within 12 hr of birth. The hepatitis B vaccine induces protective antibodies in newborns who receive the recommended three doses. HBIG provides a high titer of antibody to hepatitis B surface antigen. The vaccine provides prophylaxis against infection of newborns born to mothers who carry or are infected with hepatitis B.

(N) **NCLEX® Connection: Health Promotion and Maintenance, Health Promotion/Disease Prevention**

3. A nurse is providing care to a newborn after birth. Which of the following mechanisms will prevent heat loss from convection? (Select all that apply.)

	Drying the newborn after delivery
X	**Placing a cap over the newborn's head**
X	**Swaddling the newborn**
X	**Placing the newborn in the radiant warmer**
X	**Placing the newborn's bassinet away from a fan**

   To prevent heat loss from convection, use a blanket to swaddle the newborn and keep the newborn's head covered. Perform procedures under a radiant heat source. The newborn's bassinet should be positioned out of the direct line of a fan or air conditioning vent. Drying the newborn immediately following delivery prevents heat loss through evaporation. Evaporation is the loss of heat that occurs when a liquid is converted to a vapor. In a newborn, heat loss by evaporation occurs as a result of vaporization of the moisture from the skin.

(N) **NCLEX® Connection: Health Promotion and Maintenance, Ante/Intra/Postpartum and Newborn Care**

4. A nurse is providing care for a newborn after birth. Which of the following nursing actions is the highest priority?

    A. Initiating breastfeeding

    B. Determining the newborn's gestational age

    C. Administering a vitamin K injection

    D. Covering the newborn's head with a cap

    The greatest risk to the newborn is cold stress. Therefore, the highest priority intervention is to prevent heat loss. Covering a newborn's head with a cap prevents cold stress due to excessive evaporative heat loss. Initiating breastfeeding is important following birth, but it is not the priority. Performing a gestational age assessment is important, but it is not the priority intervention. Vitamin K can be given immediately after birth, but it is not the highest priority.

NCLEX® Connection: Health Promotion and Maintenance, Ante/Intra/Postpartum and Newborn Care

5. A charge nurse is educating a newly licensed nurse regarding the administration of vitamin K (Aquamephyton) to a newborn. Which of the following is an appropriate response by the nurse to include in the teaching?

    A. "Vitamin K provides immunity."

    B. "Vitamin K assists with blood clotting."

    C. "Vitamin K assists the bowel in maturing."

    D. "Vitamin K prevents cold stress."

Vitamin K is deficient in a newborn because the colon is sterile. For vitamin K to be produced, there must be bacteria available. Once a newborn receives the first feeding, the bacteria will be produced. Until that point, a newborn is at risk of hemorrhagic disease. Vitamin K is required to activate clotting factors II, VII, IX, and X. Vitamin K does not provide immunity, assist the bowel in maturing, or prevent cold stress.

NCLEX® Connection: Health Promotion and Maintenance, Ante/Intra/Postpartum and Newborn Care

6. A nurse is transporting a newborn to his mother following a circumcision. Which of the following security actions should the nurse take?

    A. Validate the newborn's security tag number with the mother's number.

    B. Ask the mother to identify the newborn.

    C. Match the mother's identification band with the newborn's.

    D. Compare the newborn's name on the identification band with the crib card.

The mother, newborn, and significant other are identified by plastic identification wristbands with permanent locks that must be cut to be removed. Identification bands should include the newborn's name and sex, and date and time of birth. Each time a newborn is taken to the parents, the identification band should be verified against the mother's identification band. Validating the newborn's security tag number, asking the mother to identify the newborn, and comparing the newborn's name on the crib card to the identification band are not correct security actions the nurse should take.

 NCLEX® Connection: Safety and Infection Control, Security Plan

7. A nurse is reinforcing teaching to a mother regarding breastfeeding. Which of the following actions by the mother indicates the need for additional teaching?

    A. The mother expresses a few drops of colostrum and places it on her nipple.

    B. The mother inserts a finger in the side of the newborn's mouth before removing the nipple from the newborn's mouth.

    C. The mother gently strokes the newborn's lips with her nipple when she is ready to breastfeed.

    D. The mother places a breast shield over her nipple before placing the nipple in the newborn's mouth.

A breast shield is not routinely used for breastfeeding. A breast shield is worn when the nipples are flat or inverted, or occasionally when they are sore and cracked. All the other techniques are appropriate for breastfeeding.

 NCLEX® Connection: Health Promotion and Maintenance, Ante/Intra/Postpartum and Newborn Care

8. A nurse is reinforcing teaching to a mother about proper techniques for bottle feeding. Which of the following statements made by the mother indicates an understanding of the teaching?

    A. "I will burp my baby at the end of the feeding."

    B. "I should hold my baby close in a supine position."

    C. "I will keep the nipple full of formula throughout the feeding."

    D. "I should refrigerate any unused formula."

The nipple should always be kept full of formula to prevent the newborn from sucking in air during the feeding. The newborn should be burped after each ½ oz and should be cradled in a semi-upright position. Any unused formula should be discarded due to the possibility of bacterial contamination.

NCLEX® Connection: Health Promotion and Maintenance, Ante/Intra/Postpartum and Newborn Care

9. A nurse is aware that which of the following is a contraindication for circumcising a male newborn? (Select all that apply.)

    | __X__ | **Hypospadias** |
    | _____ | Hydrocele |
    | __X__ | **Familiar history of hemophilia** |
    | _____ | Hyperbilirubinemia |
    | __X__ | **Epispadias** |

    In hypospadias and epispadias, the urethra is located somewhere other than the tip of the urethra, and the foreskin is needed for plastic surgery to repair the defect. Familiar history of bleeding disorders, hypospadias, and epispadias are all contraindications for circumcision of a newborn. Hydrocele and hyperbilirubinemia are not contraindications.

    Ⓝ NCLEX® Connection: Reduction of Risk Potential, Potential for Complications of Diagnostic Tests/Treatments/Procedures

10. A nurse is reinforcing discharge teaching to the parents of a newborn. Which of the following statements made by the parents requires additional education?

    A. "I should keep my baby's cord dry and clean with the diaper folded below it."

    B. "I will not remove the yellow exudate that will form on my baby's circumcision."

    C. "I will place my baby's car seat in the back seat in a semi-reclined, rear-facing position."

    D. "I should give my baby some water until my breast milk comes in."

    Infants who weigh up to 9.1 kg (20 lb) should be restrained in a car seat in a semi-reclined, rear-facing position in the back seat of the car. The newborn's cord should be kept dry and clean to help reduce infection and hasten drying. Folding the diaper below the cord prevents urine from the diaper penetrating the cord site. Yellow exudate that forms on the circumcision should not be removed. Newborns should not be given water supplements because they receive enough water from breast milk. Thus, this response requires additional education by the nurse.

    Ⓝ NCLEX® Connection: Safety and Infection Control, Accident Prevention

11. A nurse is educating a mother about the proper use of the bulb syringe. Which of the following responses should the nurse include in the teaching?

   A. "Suction the baby's mouth before her nose."

   B. "Suction the baby's nose before her mouth."

   C. "Place the bulb syringe to the back of the baby's throat."

   D. "Compress the syringe after it is placed in the baby's mouth or nose."

   When suctioning the newborn with a bulb syringe, the bulb should be compressed before it is placed in the newborn's mouth or nose. The newborn's mouth should be suctioned before the nose to prevent aspiration during the gasp response. Also, the back of the newborn's throat should not be touched when suctioning the mouth because the gag reflex may be stimulated. The bulb syringe should be compressed before inserting it into the newborn's mouth.

   Ⓝ **NCLEX® Connection: Health Promotion and Maintenance, Ante/Intra/Postpartum and Newborn Care**

UNIT 4	NEWBORN NURSING CARE
Chapter 15	Complications of the Newborn

Overview

- Newborns may experience complications following birth. Often, data collection findings are not specific and it may be difficult to identify the cause. Complications may be discovered during routine care of newborns. Complications include prematurity, small-for-gestational-age (SGA) newborn, large-for-gestational-age (LGA)/macrosomic newborn, postterm newborn, respiratory distress syndrome, substance withdrawal, fetal alcohol syndrome, infection, cold stress, and hypoglycemia.

Risk Factors

MATERNAL RISK FACTORS	NEONATAL RISK FACTORS
• Diabetes mellitus	• Prematurity, postmaturity
• Epidural anesthesia	• LGA, SGA
• Use of barbiturates or narcotics close to birth	• Stress at birth, such as cold stress and asphyxia (meconium staining, cord prolapse, and nuchal cord)
• Bleeding disorders	
• Gestational hypertension	• Congenital or chromosomal anomalies
• Multiple pregnancies	• Infection
• Adolescent pregnancy	• Genetic factors
• Lack of prenatal care	• Rh- or ABO-incompatibility
• Smoking	
• Preterm labor, previous history of preterm delivery	
• Abnormalities of the uterus	
• Cervical incompetence	
• Premature rupture of the membranes	
• Infections – TORCH, UTI, HIV	
• Maternal substance abuse	

- Objective Data

  - Physical assessment findings

    - Prematurity – A newborn born after 20 weeks of gestation and before 37 weeks of gestation is considered a preterm newborn. Preterm newborns are at risk for a variety of complications due to immature organ systems including RDS, bronchopulmonary dysplasia, aspiration, intraventricular hemorrhage, retinopathy of prematurity, patent ductus arteriosus, and necrotizing enterocolitis (NEC).

      - A Ballard assessment shows a physical and neurological assessment totaling less than 37 weeks of gestation.

      - Signs of increased respiratory effort and/or respiratory distress include nasal flaring or retractions of the chest wall during inspirations; expiratory grunting; tachypnea; periods of apnea longer than 10 to 15 seconds; and periodic breathing consisting of 5- to 10-second respiratory pauses, followed by 10 to 15-second compensatory rapid respirations.

      - Low birth weight with large head in comparison to total body size

      - Minimal subcutaneous fat deposit with wrinkled features

      - Weak reflexes including grasp, suck, swallow, gag and cough

      - Hypotonic muscles, decreased level of activity, lethargy, and a weak cry

    - Small for gestational age (SGA) describes newborns whose birth weight is at or below the 10th percentile. Common complications of infants who are SGA are perinatal asphyxia, meconium aspiration, hypoglycemia, polycythemia, and instability of body temperature.

      - Weight below 10th percentile, normal skull, but reduced body dimensions

      - Wide skull sutures from inadequate bone growth

      - Dry, loose skin, decreased subcutaneous fat, decreased muscle mass, particularly over the cheeks and buttocks

      - Thin, dry, yellow, and dull umbilical cord rather than gray, glistening, and moist

      - Hypotonia

    - Large for gestational age (LGA) or macrosomia, describes newborns whose birth weight is above the 90th percentile or more than 4,000 g (8 lb, 12 oz). LGA newborns are at risk for birth injuries (shoulder dystocia, clavicle fracture or a cesarean birth, asphyxia, hypoglycemia, polycythemia and Erb-Duchenne paralysis due to birth trauma).

      - Weight above 90th percentile (4,000 g)

      - Plump and full-faced (cushingoid appearance) from increased subcutaneous fat

      - Signs of hypoxia including tachypnea, retractions, cyanosis, nasal flaring, and grunting

- □ Birth trauma (fractures, intracranial hemorrhage, and CNS injury)
- □ Sluggishness, hypotonic muscles, and hypoactivity
- ■ Postterm newborn
  - □ Wasted appearance, thin with loose skin, having lost some of the subcutaneous fat. Most of the vernix has been lost.
  - □ Peeling, cracked, and dry skin; leathery from decreased protection of vernix and amniotic fluid
  - □ Long, thin body
  - □ Meconium staining of fingernails and umbilical cord
  - □ Hair and nails may be long
  - □ Macrosomia
- ○ Laboratory tests
  - ■ Blood glucose
    - □ Confirmation of hypoglycemia – Two consecutive serum glucose levels less than 40 mg/dL in a newborn who is term, and less than 25 mg/dL in a newborn who is preterm
  - ■ Culture and sensitivity of the blood, urine, and cerebrospinal fluid, positive blood cultures, usually polymicrobial (more than one pathogen) indicates the presence of infection/sepsis
  - ■ Serum bilirubin – Direct and indirect
  - ■ A direct Coombs test reveals the presence of antibody-coated (sensitized) Rh-positive RBCs in the newborn.
  - ■ CBC – May show polycythemia (Hct greater than 65%) from in-utero hypoxia
    - □ A maternal and newborn blood type is done to determine if there is a presence of ABO incapability. This occurs if the newborn has blood type A, B, or AB, and the mother is type O.
  - ■ Serum electrolytes
    - □ Serum calcium – Hypocalcemia from long and difficult birth
  - ■ Drug screen of urine to identify suspected maternal drug use.
- ○ Diagnostic procedures
  - ■ ABGs
  - ■ Chest x-ray to rule out meconium aspiration syndrome, congenital heart defects

Collaborative Care

- • Nursing Care for All Newborns
  - ○ Monitor vital signs, I&O, and daily weight.
  - ○ Observe skin turgor, mucous membranes, and fontanels for signs of dehydration.

○ Provide adequate nutrition

○ Initiate early feedings.

○ Monitor the newborn's ability to suck, swallow, and digest nutrients.

○ Administer frequent, small feedings of high-calorie formula – May need gavage feedings.

○ Maintain adequate hydration.

○ Elevate the infant's head during and following feedings, and burp him/her to reduce vomiting and aspiration.

○ Have suction available to reduce the risk for aspiration.

○ Provide a neutral thermal environment for newborns (isolette or radiant heat warmer) to prevent cold stress.

○ Provide skin and mouth care.

○ Observe the newborn's behavior.

○ Reduce external stimuli. Touch newborns very smoothly and lightly. Keep lighting dim and noise levels reduced.

   ■ Cluster nursing care. Provide care to conserve the newborn's energy.

      □ Swaddle newborns to reduce self-stimulation and protect the skin from abrasions.

      □ For newborns who are addicted to cocaine, use vertical rocking and a pacifier.

○ Monitor newborns for bleeding from puncture sites and the gastrointestinal tract.

○ Administer oxygen as prescribed.

○ Monitor newborns receiving IV fluids

○ Provide for nonnutritive sucking, such as using a pacifier while gavage feeding.

○ Protect newborns against infection by using standard precautions, performing hand hygiene and using gowns. Provide individualized equipment for newborns such as a thermometer and stethoscope.

○ Support respiratory efforts and suction the newborn as necessary to maintain an open airway.

○ Monitor the newborn's visitors for infection.

RESPIRATORY DISTRESS SYNDROME

Overview

- Respiratory distress syndrome (RDS) occurs as a result of surfactant deficiency in the lungs and is characterized by poor gas exchange and ventilatory failure.

  o Objective Data

    ▪ Physical assessment findings

      □ Tachypnea (respiratory rate greater than 60/min)

      □ Nasal flaring

      □ Expiratory grunting

      □ Intercostal and substernal retractions

      □ Labored breathing

      □ Fine rales on auscultation

      □ Cyanosis

      □ Unresponsiveness, flaccidity, and apnea with decreased breath sounds (clinical manifestations of worsened RDS)

Collaborative Care

- Suction the infant's mouth, trachea, and nose as needed.

- Maintain thermoregulation.

- Provide mouth and skin care.

NEONATAL SUBSTANCE WITHDRAWAL

Overview

- Substance withdrawal in the newborn occurs when the mother uses drugs that have addictive properties during pregnancy. This includes illegal drugs, alcohol, tobacco, and prescription drugs. Newborns may experience withdrawal symptoms from substances or fetal alcohol syndrome (FAS), which results from the chronic or periodic intake of alcohol during pregnancy.

Data Collection

- o Objective data
  - ■ Physical assessment findings
    - □ CNS – Increased wakefulness, sleep pattern disturbances, a high-pitched, shrill cry, incessant crying, irritability, tremors, hyperactive, may have an increased or decreased Moro reflex, hypersensitivity to sound and external stimuli, increased deep-tendon reflexes, increased muscle tone, abrasions and/or excoriations on the face and knees, and seizures.
    - □ Metabolic, vasomotor, and respiratory findings – Nasal congestion with flaring, frequent yawning, skin mottling, tachypnea greater than 60/min, sweating, hypothermia or hyperthermia.
    - □ Gastrointestinal – Poor feeding, poor weight gain, dehydration, regurgitation (projectile vomiting), diarrhea, and excessive, uncoordinated, and constant sucking.
  - ■ Fetal Alcohol Syndrome
    - □ Objective data
      - ▸ Physical assessment findings
        - ▷ Facial anomalies include eyes with epicanthal folds, strabismus, and ptosis; mouth with a poor suck, small teeth, and cleft lip or palate
        - ▷ Deafness
        - ▷ Abnormal palmar creases and irregular hair
        - ▷ Many vital organ anomalies, such as heart defects, including atrial and ventricular septal defects, tetralogy of Fallot, and patent-ductus arteriosus
        - ▷ Developmental delays and neurologic abnormalities
        - ▷ Prenatal and postnatal growth retardation
        - ▷ Sleep disturbances

Collaborative Care

- • Monitor the newborn's ability to feed and digest intake.
- • Monitor the newborn's fluids and electrolytes such as skin turgor, mucous membranes, fontanels, and I&O.
- • Observe the infant's behavior.

NEONATAL INFECTION/SEPSIS (SEPSIS NEONATORUM)

(@) Overview

- Infection may be contracted by newborns before, during, or after delivery. Neonatal sepsis is the presence of microorganisms or their toxins in the blood or tissues of the infant during the first month after birth. Organisms frequently responsible for neonatal infections include: Staphylococcus aureus, S. epidermidis, Escherichia coli, Haemophilus influenzae, and streptococcus ß-hemolytic, Group B.

  o Neonatal infection/sepsis (Sepsis Neonatorum)

  o Objective data

    ■ Physical assessment findings

      □ Temperature instability

      □ Suspicious drainage (eyes, umbilical stump)

      □ Poor feeding pattern, such as a weak suck or decreased intake

      □ Vomiting and diarrhea

      □ Poor weight gain

      □ Abdominal distention, large residual if feeding by gavage

      □ Apnea, sternal retractions, grunting, and nasal flaring

      □ Decreased oxygen saturation

      □ Color changes such as pallor, jaundice, and petechiae

      □ Tachycardia or bradycardia

      □ Tachypnea

      □ Low blood pressure

      □ Irritability and seizure activity

      □ Poor muscle tone and lethargic

COLD STRESS

(@) Overview

- Cold stress (complication of ineffective thermoregulation) can lead to hypoxia, acidosis, and hypoglycemia. Newborns with RDS are at a higher risk for hypothermia.

  o Objective data

    ■ Physical assessment findings

      □ Drop in temperature is first sign

      □ Respiratory rate starts to increase and then apneic spells occur

□ Heart rate starts to increase and then is followed by bradycardia

□ Skin appears mottled with acrocyanosis that may become cyanotic

□ Physical activity is dependent on respiratory distress. Respiratory distress causes newborns to have decreased activity, whereas increased activity occurs with newborns who do not have respiratory distress.

Collaborative Care

- Check the newborn's axillary temperature every hour until it becomes stable.

- Report an axillary temperature of less than 36.5° C (97.7° F).

- If temperature is unstable, place newborns in a radiant warmer and maintain skin temperature at approximately 36.5° C (97.7° F).

- Perform all procedures on newborns under a radiant warmer. Practice techniques to minimize heat loss (warm equipment before placing on the newborn's skin, keep bassinets away from windows).

- If cold stress does occur, warm newborns slowly over a period of 2 to 4 hr, administer oxygen and provide for feeding to prevent hypoglycemia.

- Medications

  o Phenobarbital (Solfoton)

    ■ Anticonvulsant to decrease CNS irritability and control seizures for newborns who have alcohol or opioid addiction.

    ■ Nursing considerations

      □ Monitor newborns for seizure activity.

  o Beractant (Survanta)

    ■ Lung surfactant to manage RDS and improve respiratory status

  o Betamethasone (Celestone)

    ■ Glucocorticoids are administered for a 24-hr period prior to delivery to promote fetal lung development and increase surfactant in an attempt to prevent RDS.

  o Ampicillin (Principen)

    ■ Antibiotic used for broad-spectrum bactericidal effect

    ■ Nursing considerations

      □ Ensure blood cultures have been obtained prior to administration of antibiotics.

  o Gentamicin sulfate (Garamycin)

    ■ Aminoglycoside antibiotic

    ■ Nursing Considerations

      □ Ensure blood cultures have been obtained prior to administration of antibiotics.

- o   Interdisciplinary care

  - ▪   Request referral for home health nursing care.

  - ▪   Request referral for community support services.

HYPERBILIRUBINEMIA

Overview

- Hyperbilirubinemia is an elevation of serum bilirubin levels resulting in jaundice. Jaundice normally appears on the head (especially the sclera and mucous membranes), and then progresses down the thorax, abdomen, and extremities.

- Jaundice can be either physiologic or pathologic.

  - o   Physiologic jaundice is considered benign (resulting from normal newborn physiology of increased bilirubin production due to the shortened lifespan and breakdown of fetal RBCs and liver immaturity). The infant with physiologic jaundice has no other symptoms and shows signs of jaundice after 24 hr of age.

  - o   Pathologic jaundice is a result of an underlying disease. Pathologic jaundice appears before 24 hr of age or is persistent after day 7. In the term infant, bilirubin levels increase more than 0.5 mg/dL/hr, peaks at greater than 13 mg/dL, or is associated with anemia and hepatosplenomegaly. Pathologic jaundice is usually caused by a blood group incompatibility or an infection, but may be the result of RBC disorders.

- Kernicterus (bilirubin encephalopathy) can result from untreated hyperbilirubinemia with bilirubin levels at or higher than 25 mg/dL. Bilirubin deposits in brain cells may lead to cerebral palsy, epilepsy, or mental retardation.

- Objective Data

  - ▪   Physical assessment findings

    - ▫   Blanching of skin on cheek or abdomen will reveal yellowish tint to skin. Sclera and mucous membranes may also have yellowish tint.

    - ▫   Signs and symptoms of kernicterus

      - ▸   Very yellowish or orange skin

      - ▸   Lethargy

      - ▸   Hypotonic

      - ▸   Poor suck reflex

      - ▸   Increased sleepiness

      - ▸   If untreated, the infant will become hypertonic with backward arching of the neck and trunk

      - ▸   High-pitched cry

      - ▸   Fever

Collaborative Care

- Set up phototherapy if prescribed. It is prescribed if an infant's serum bilirubin is greater than 15 mg/dL prior to 48 hr of age, greater than 18 mg/dL prior to 72 hr of age, and greater than 20 mg/dL at anytime.

  ○ Place an eye mask over the newborn's eyes after they are gently closed to protect the corneas and retinas. Ensure the nares are not covered.

  ○ Keep newborns undressed except for a surgical mask placed (make like a bikini) over the genitalia to prevent possible damage from heat and light waves. Be sure to remove the metal strip from the mask to prevent burning.

  ○ Avoid applying lotions or ointments to newborns because they absorb heat and can cause burns.

  ○ Remove newborns from phototherapy every 4 hr and unmask the newborn's eyes, checking for signs of inflammation or injury.

  ○ Reposition newborns every 2 hr to expose all of the body surfaces to the phototherapy lights and prevent pressure sores.

  ○ Check the lamp energy with a photometer per unit protocol.

  ○ Turn off the phototherapy lights before drawing blood for testing.

- Observe newborns for side effects of phototherapy.

  ○ Maculopapular skin rash of papules (small raised bumps) and macules (flat discolored areas of the skin) may appear. This rash is usually self-limiting.

  ○ Pressure areas

  ○ Dehydration (poor skin turgor, dry mucous membranes, decreased urinary output)

  ○ Elevated temperature

- Monitor vital signs every 4 hr.

  ○ Monitor bilirubin levels every 4 hr until the level returns to the expected reference range.

  ○ Monitor elimination, noting frequency and consistency. Frequent, loose, stools may occur due to increased gastric motility from bilirubin breakdown. Provide meticulous skin care to prevent skin breakdown in the perineal area.

  ○ Monitor urine output. Urine may have a brown or golden color.

  ○ Monitor for signs of dehydration

    ▪ Urine output less than 1 mL/kg/hr

    ▪ Urine-specific gravity more than 1.015

    ▪ Weight loss

    ▪ Dry mucous membranes

    ▪ Poor skin turgor

    ▪ Depressed fontanel

    o   Feed newborns frequently – Every 3 to 4 hr. This will promote bilirubin excretion in the stools.

    o   Continue to breastfeed the newborn. The newborn should be breastfed at least 8 to 12 times in a 24-hour period. Supplementing with formula may be prescribed. Maintain adequate fluid intake to prevent dehydration.

    o   Explain hyperbilirubinemia, its causes, diagnostic tests, and treatment to parents.

    o   Assist with the care of newborns receiving an exchange transfusion for infants who are at risk for kernicterus.

HYPOGLYCEMIA

Overview

- Hypoglycemia is a serum glucose level of less than 40 mg/dL for term newborns occurring in the first 3 days of life and less than 25 mg/dL for preterm newborns. Untreated hypoglycemia can result in seizures, brain damage, and/or death.

Risk Factors

- Maternal diabetes mellitus
- Preterm infant
- LGA or SGA
- Stress at birth, such as cold stress and asphyxia
- Maternal epidural anesthesia

Data Collection

- Objective Data
    - Physical assessment findings
        - Poor feeding
        - Jitteriness/tremors
        - Hypothermia
        - Diaphoresis
        - Weak shrill cry
        - Lethargy
        - Flaccid muscle tone
        - Seizures/coma
        - Irregular respirations
        - Cyanosis
        - Apnea

- ○ Laboratory tests and diagnostic procedures
    - ■ Two consecutive plasma glucose levels less than 40 mg/dL in a newborn who is term, and less than 25 mg/dL in a newborn who is preterm

Collaborative Care

- Obtain blood per heel stick for glucose monitoring within 2 hr of life and monitor blood glucose level per facility protocol.

- Provide frequent oral and/or gavage feedings or continuous parenteral nutrition. Encourage early breastfeeding.

- Care After Discharge
    - ○ Client education
        - ■ Reinforce proper hand hygiene and other infection control measures (the use of clean bottles and nipples for each feeding, avoiding people with acute illness).
        - ■ Provide emotional support to families.
        - ■ Encourage families to follow up with medical appointments.

- Client Outcomes
    - ○ The newborn will adapt to extrauterine life without injury.
    - ○ The newborn will gain weight.
    - ○ The newborn will not exhibit signs of seizures.
    - ○ The newborn maintains body temperature.
    - ○ The newborn is free of signs of infection.
    - ○ The newborn maintains a blood glucose level within the expected reference range.
    - ○ The newborn will display adequate oxygenation as evidenced by respiratory rate and blood gas levels within expected reference range.
    - ○ The newborn will display a serum-bilirubin level within the expected reference range.

Ⓐ APPLICATION EXERCISES

1. A nurse is called to assist with the data collection of a newborn who was born at 30 weeks of gestation. The newborn's birth weight is 1,025 g. Her Apgar scores are 2 at 1 min and 7 at 5 min. She is displaying grunting, nasal flaring, and intercostal retractions. Which of the following are characteristics of a preterm newborn that the nurse may observe? (Select all that apply.)

   _____ Large head in comparison to body

   _____ Lanugo

   _____ Lusty cry

   _____ Lethargy

   _____ Translucent skin

2. A nurse is examining a newborn who was delivered at 42 weeks of gestation. Which of the following characteristics indicates that the newborn is postterm? (Select all that apply.)

   _____ Abundant lanugo

   _____ Flat areola without breast buds

   _____ Macrosomia

   _____ Leathery skin

   _____ Peeling of the hands and feet

3. A nurse is caring for a newborn who is 36 hrs of age with a serum bilirubin of 17 mg/dL. Phototherapy is prescribed by the provider. Which of the following findings should the nurse report to the provider?

   A. Golden-colored urine

   B. Frequent loose stools

   C. Sunken fontanels

   D. Maculopapular skin rash

4. A nurse is collecting data on a newborn with a blood glucose level of 30 mg/dL. Which of the following findings require intervention?

   A. Acrocyanosis

   B. Diaphoresis

   C. Lusty cry

   D. Flexed extremities

5. A nurse should consider the possibility of neonatal withdrawal syndrome if a newborn

   A. has decreased muscle tone.

   B. has a continuous high-pitched cry.

   C. sleeps for 2 hr after feeding.

   D. has mild tremors when disturbed.

(A) APPLICATION EXERCISES ANSWER KEY

1. A nurse is called to assist with the data collection of a newborn who was born at 30 weeks of gestation. The newborn's birth weight is 1,025 g. Her Apgar scores are 2 at 1 min and 7 at 5 min. She is displaying grunting, nasal flaring, and intercostal retractions. Which of the following are characteristics of a preterm newborn that the nurse may observe? (Select all that apply.)

    __X__ **Large head in comparison to body**

    __X__ **Lanugo**

    _____ Lusty cry

    __X__ **Lethargy**

    __X__ **Translucent skin**

    Characteristics of a preterm newborn include large head in comparison to body, lanugo over the body, and skin that is thin, smooth, shiny, and may be translucent. Also, hypotonic muscle tone and lethargy is noted. A lusty cry is seen in a term newborn and preterm newborns have a weak cry.

    (N) NCLEX® Connection: Health Promotion and Maintenance, Data Collection Techniques

2. A nurse is examining a newborn who was delivered at 42 weeks of gestation. Which of the following characteristics indicates that the newborn is postterm? (Select all that apply.)

    _____ Abundant lanugo

    _____ Flat areola without breast buds

    __X__ **Macrosomia**

    __X__ **Leathery skin**

    __X__ **Peeling of the hands and feet**

    Leathery, cracked, and wrinkled skin is seen in a postterm newborn due to placental insufficiency. Additionally, peeling of the hands and feet are noted. Macrosomia is also characteristic of the postterm newborn. Abundant lanugo and flat areolas without breast buds are found in preterm newborns.

    (N) NCLEX® Connection: Physiological Adaptation, Alterations in Body Systems

3. A nurse is caring for a newborn who is 36 hrs of age with a serum bilirubin of 17 mg/dL. Phototherapy is prescribed by the provider. Which of the following findings should the nurse report to the provider?

   A. Golden-colored urine

   B. Frequent loose stools

   C. Sunken fontanels

   D. Maculopapular skin rash

   Infants receiving phototherapy are at greatest risk for dehydration related to the loss of water from frequent loose stools due to increased bilirubin excretion. Supplemental oral or intravenous fluids are given as needed to prevent the complication. Golden-colored urine, frequent loose stools, and maculopapular rash are all findings that may be seen in the newborn receiving phototherapy. However, these do not warrant notification of the provider.

 NCLEX® Connection: Physiological Adaptation, Alterations in Body Systems

4. A nurse is collecting data on a newborn with a blood glucose level of 30 mg/dL. Which of the following findings require intervention?

   A. Acrocyanosis

   B. Diaphoresis

   C. Lusty cry

   D. Flexed extremities

   Physical assessment findings associated with hypoglycemia include diaphoresis, poor feeding, jitteriness, hypothermia, weak high-pitched cry, lethargy, flaccid muscle tone, eye rolling, seizures, irregular respirations, cyanosis, and apnea. Acrocyanosis, lusty cry, and flexed extremities are normal findings seen in the newborn.

 NCLEX® Connection: Physiological Adaptation, Alterations in Body Systems

5. A nurse should consider the possibility of neonatal withdrawal syndrome if a newborn

   A. has decreased muscle tone.

   B. has a continuous high-pitched cry.

   C. sleeps for 2 hr after feeding.

   D. has mild tremors when disturbed.

   Symptoms of withdrawal from maternal substance abuse include an excessive or continuous high-pitched cry, and a markedly hyperactive Moro reflex. A newborn withdrawing from opioids or other substances abused maternally is likely to have an increased muscle tone along with other central nervous system disturbances. Most newborns sleep for varying amounts of time after feeding. Symptoms of withdrawal from maternal substance abuse include difficulty moving through various sleep stages. The sleep pattern disturbance is related to central nervous system excitation secondary to drug or alcohol withdrawal. Many newborns have mild tremors when they are disturbed. What distinguishes infants who have neonatal abstinence syndrome from this normal pattern is that they have moderate to severe tremors when they are undisturbed.

 NCLEX® Connection: Health Promotion and Maintenance, Data Collection Techniques

References

Dudek, S. G. (2010). *Nutrition essentials for nursing practice* (6th ed.). Philadelphia: Lippincott Williams & Wilkins.

Grodner, M., Long, S., & Walkingshaw, B. C. (2007). *Foundations and clinical applications of nutrition: A nursing approach* (4th ed.). St. Louis, MO: Mosby.

Hockenberry, M. J., & Wilson, D. (2009). *Wong's essentials of pediatric nursing* (8th ed.). St. Louis, MO: Mosby.

Lehne, R. A. (2010). *Pharmacology for nursing care* (7th ed.). St. Louis: Saunders.

Lowdermilk, D. L., & Perry, S. E. (2007). *Maternity & women's health care* (9th ed.). St. Louis, MO: Mosby.

Perry, S., Hockenberry, M., Lowdermilk, D., Wilson, D. (2010). *Maternal child nursing care* (4th ed.). Maryland Heights, MO: Mosby.

Pillitteri, A. (2007). *Maternal and child health nursing: Care of the childbearing and childrearing family* (5th ed.). Philadelphia: Lippincott Williams & Wilkins.

Wilson, B. A., Shannon, M. T., & Shields, K. M. (2011). *Pearson nurse's drug guide 2011*. Upper Saddle River, NJ: Pearson.